AF556690

INVERSE AND ILL-POSED PROBLEMS SERIES

Uniqueness Questions in Reconstruction of Multidimensional Objects from Tomography-Type Projection Data

Also available in the Inverse and Ill-Posed Problems Series:

Monte Carlo Method for Solving Inverse Problems of Radiation Transfer
V.S. Antyufeev

Introduction to the Theory of Inverse Problems
A.L. Bukhgeim

Identification Problems of Wave Phenomena - Theory and Numerics
S.I. Kabanikhin and A. Lorenzi

Inverse Problems of Electromagnetic Geophysical Fields
P.S. Martyshko

Composite Type Equations and Inverse Problems
A.I. Kozhanov

Inverse Problems of Vibrational Spectroscopy
A.G. Yagola, I.V. Kochikov, G.M. Kuramshina and Yu.A. Pentin

Elements of the Theory of Inverse Problems
A.M. Denisov

Volterra Equations and Inverse Problems
A.L. Bughgeim

Small Parameter Method in Multidimensional Inverse Problems
A.S. Barashkov

Regularization, Uniqueness and Existence of Volterra Equations of the First Kind
A. Asanov

Methods for Solution of Nonlinear Operator Equations
V.P. Tanana

Inverse and Ill-Posed Sources Problems
Yu.E. Anikonov, B.A. Bubnov and G.N. Erokhin

Methods for Solving Operator Equations
V.P. Tanana

Nonclassical and Inverse Problems for Pseudoparabolic Equations
A. Asanov and E.R. Atamanov

Formulas in Inverse and Ill-Posed Problems
Yu.E. Anikonov

Inverse Logarithmic Potential Problem
V.G. Cherednichenko

Multidimensional Inverse and Ill-Posed Problems for Differential Equations
Yu.E. Anikonov

Ill-Posed Problems with A Priori Information
V.V. Vasin and A.L. Ageev

Integral Geometry of Tensor Fields
V.A. Sharafutdinov

Inverse Problems for Maxwell's Equations
V.G. Romanov and S.I. Kabanikhin

INVERSE AND ILL-POSED PROBLEMS SERIES

Uniqueness Questions in Reconstruction of Multidimensional Objects from Tomography-Type Projection Data

V.P. Golubyatnikov

///VSP///

UTRECHT • BOSTON • KÖLN • TOKYO

2000

VSP BV
P.O. Box 346
3700 AH Zeist
The Netherlands

Tel: +31 30 692 57
Fax: +31 30 693 20
vsppub@compuserve.co
www.vsppub.cc

First published in 2000

ISBN 90-6764-332-7

Printed in The Netherlands by Ridderprint bv, Ridderkerk.

Contents

Preface

A wide class of problems in various domains of pure, applied and industrial mathematics can be formulated as follows:

How can one determine the structure or just the shape of a "Black Box" from a collection of the "Input-Output" measurements?

Or in the following analytical form:

Given the initial and the terminal states of a system, how can one determine the evolution equation of a special type, which describes the behavior of the system, its geometrical and other characteristics?

Inverse problems of this type appear in different domains of applied mathematics and physics: in location, multichannel measurements in the inverse problems of diffraction and other fields of wave optics (see Aben, 1979; Antsiferov *et al.* , 1997; Kireitov, 1983), in tomography (Natterer, 1986; Sharafutdinov, 1992), in seismology (Čherveny *et al.* , 1977; Gol'din, 1997) and in the theory of differential equations (Anikonov, 1995a). Each of these domains has its own preferable representation of the "Input-Output" data.

One of the most well-known practical and, at the same time, theoretical examples of problem of this type is that of determination of the shape of a (convex) body from the shapes of its projections.

In the first three chapters of this book we study the uniqueness questions of recovering the shapes of the convex and more complicated bodies from the shapes of their projections onto the planes of low dimensions. We obtain some stability estimates of the solutions to these inverse problems.

Similar classical inverse problems in the geometrical optics approximation have been studied in the mathematical literature from different viewpoints (see, for example, Aleksandrov, 1937; Pogorelov, 1973; Gel'fand *et al.* , 1980; Bonnesen and Fenchel, 1987).

In many publications devoted to these problems, the "Output" data are represented by the sections of the multidimensional objects, not their projections (see Gardner, 1980, 1992, 1995; Montejano, 1991), but in some interesting cases the procedure of the polar duality allows reducing the corresponding problems to the problems with the "Output" data of projection type.

In Chapter 4 we study some inverse problems with the projection data directly connected with tomography, in particular, with the apparent contours of the smooth surfaces, which have many useful practical interpretations: thin cracks in continuous media which are studied in industrial defectoscopy, the caustic surfaces which are studied in wave optics, etc. We formulate some sufficient conditions of coincidence of the shapes of two hypersurfaces, if the shapes of their apparent contours on any 2-dimensional plane coincide. Here we obtain also some new results on reconstruction of smooth surfaces from observations of the wave fronts generated by these surfaces. We derive new explicit inversion formulae for the integral geometry problems similar to those obtained in the local case in Gel'fand *et al.* (1967).

The main goal of the second part of Chapter 4 is to study inverse problems for the Hamilton – Jacobi equations and for the evolution equations of another special type. We construct the explicit formulae for the solutions to these problems from the "Input-Output" information on the endpoints of the trajectories of the corresponding Hamiltonian system (Section 4.3) and trajectories of the action of an operator semigroup (Section 4.4). Both of these constructions are typical for the tomographic investigations.

Preface

I would like to express my sincere gratitude to the chiefs and all participants of the geometry seminar of A. D. Aleksandrov and the seminar of Yu. E. Anikonov for stimulating discussions, critical notes, advice and helpful assistance, which constantly accompanied my work since 1977. I am, especially, indebted to Natalie Ayupova, Vladimir Ionin, Valerii Kireitov, Aleksandr Kuz'minykh, Victor Toponogov, Dmitrii Trotsenko and Vladimir Sharafutdinov.

Many useful suggestions I have got during my meetings with Yurii Adamchik, Lev Aizenberg, Stefano Campi, Yakov Eliashberg, Richard Gardner, Sergei Gol'din, Victor Palamodov, Vadim Seleznev, Iskander Taimanov, Alesha Volčič and Yosif Yomdin.

A special *Vielen Dank* is addressed to Helmut Groemer who has discovered a mistake in one of my first publications on the reconstruction problems (see Groemer, 1987).

The work was supported by Russian Foundation for the Basic Research, grant No. 99-01–00607.

Vladimir Golubyatnikov

Chapter 1.

Introduction

The main results of the first part of this book concern a classical question: if two convex bodies in the Euclidean space $\mathbb{R}^3$ have congruent projections onto any plane, how different shapes can they have? The same question can be posed for the higher-dimensional spaces $\mathbb{R}^n$ and for the complex Euclidean spaces, which we shall denote by $\mathbb{C}^n$ (note that sometimes, see Chakerian and Groemer (1983), this symbol signifies the class of all convex compact bodies in $\mathbb{R}^n$). The most general statement of this **Main Question** seems as follows:

MQ: *Let V_1 and V_2 be compact convex bodies in the n-dimensional Euclidean space and let their orthogonal projections onto any k-dimensional plane be transformable into each other by some linear automorphism of the k-dimensional Euclidean space. How different can these convex (or more intricate) compact bodies be? Which transformations of the ambient space can transform these bodies into each other?*

Various problems related to this question have been studied in the literature from different viewpoints.

In connection with this question and some of its analogues, Richard Gardner and the author formulated the following puzzle about the "continual Rubik's cube" (Golubyatnikov, 1995a):

Let f and g be continuous functions defined on S^m, $m > 1$, and let their restrictions on any great circle E of this sphere coincide after some rotation $\varphi(E)$ of this circle:

$$f(\omega) = g(\varphi(E)(\omega)); \quad \omega \in E.$$

Is it true that $f(\omega) = g(\omega)$ or $f(\omega) = g(-\omega)$ for all $\omega \in S^m$? For the even functions $f(\omega) = f(-\omega)$ and $g(\omega) = g(-\omega)$ on the two-dimensional sphere the positive answer is well known (Blaschke, 1949).

Many publications were devoted to the reconstruction of convex, star and other bodies from the numerical projection data, such as the areas of shadows, the perimeters or areas of their sections and projections, etc. See, for example, Aleksandrov (1937), Chakerian (1970), Pogorelov (1973), Anikonov (1969), Anikonov and Stepanov (1981), Ball (1991), Campi (1986), Gardner and Volčič (1994b), Gel'fand *et al.* (1980). We shall give the corresponding citations below, large majority of them were mentioned in the nice geometric monograph Gardner (1995).

1.1. NOTATION AND BASIC DEFINITIONS

As is adopted in the literature, a **convex body** in a finite-dimensional vector space will be defined as a compact convex set with interior points (see, for example, Chakerian and Groemer, 1983; Gardner, 1995). In the sequel we shall assume that $n > 2$ and all the projections of the objects under consideration are orthogonal. When we do not care of the scalars, we shall denote the n-dimensional Euclidean and vector spaces by $\mathbf{E}^n$, i. e., in the real, complex and quaternionic cases at once.

Most of the notations and definitions listed below are well known and will be discussed thoroughly whenever it will be necessary. However, we shall recall some of them right now.

Definition 1.1.1. S^{n-1} denotes the unit sphere in the real Euclidean space $\mathbb{R}^n$. Let $P(\omega)$ be the oriented hyperplane in $\mathbb{R}^n$ containing the origin of the space $\mathbb{R}^n$ and orthogonal to a unit vector $\omega \in S^{n-1}$. The intersection $S^{n-2} = S^{n-1} \cap P(\omega)$ will be called a *great* $(n-2)$*-dimensional sphere.* We shall denote by $W(\omega)$ the projection of a set $W \subset \mathbb{R}^n$ onto the hyperplane $P(\omega)$. In a similar way, for a k-dimensional plane $P^k \subset \mathbb{R}^n$, $k < n-1$, we shall denote by $W(P^k)$ the orthogonal projection of $W \subset \mathbb{R}^n$ onto the plane P^k.

Definition 1.1.2. Given a convex compact body V in a Euclidean space $\mathbf{E}$, we shall denote by $H(\omega)$ or $h(\omega)$ the *support function* of V: $H(\omega) = \max\limits_{X \in V}\langle X, \omega\rangle$, where $\omega \in \mathbf{E}$ is a unit vector and $\langle\cdot,\cdot\rangle$ is the scalar product in $\mathbf{E}$. Usually, we shall consider the support functions of convex bodies with respect to the origin O of the space $\mathbf{E}$ as in the formula above. Here the points $X, Y \ldots$ in the vector space are identified with the vectors OX, OY, etc. and we shall use the common notation λV for the set of points $\{\lambda X \mid X \in V\}$ in a vector space.

Definition 1.1.3. For a unit vector $\omega \in \mathbf{E}$ and for a compact convex body V, we shall denote by $w(\omega) = H(\omega) + H(-\omega)$ the *width function* of V in the direction of this vector, i. e., the distance between the support planes to this convex body V that perpendicular to ω.

Given a compact set A in a Euclidean space, the maximal distance between points of A is called the *diameter* of A.

It is well known, that for a convex compact body its diameter coincides with the maximum of its width function.

Definition 1.1.4. We shall call a compact body $W \subset \mathbf{E}^n$ in n-dimensional vector space *k-visible* if each $(k-m)$-dimensional plane which is disjoint from W is contained in some k-dimensional plane that is disjoint from W as well. Here $0 < m \leq k < n$, and the zero-dimensional plane is a point.

Definition 1.1.5. We shall call a compact body $W \subset \mathbf{E}^n$ in n-dimensional vector space *k-convex* if for every point $x \notin W$ there is a k-dimensional plane that contains x and is disjoint from W.

In complex analysis the complements to the k-convex compact bodies in $\mathbb{C}^n$ are often called $(n-k-1)$-linearly concave domains (Aizenberg and Yuzhakov, 1979). Similar definitions can be given in the case of projective spaces as well, see Gel'fand *et al.* (1980), Znamenskii (1985), etc.

It is easy to verify that:

- a connected $(n-1)$-visible compact body in $\mathbb{R}^n$ is convex;
- projections of q-visible compact body onto any hyperplane are $(q-1)$-visible, in particular, projections of $(n-2)$-visible body in $\mathbb{R}^n$ onto any 3-dimensional plane are 1-visible, or, equivalently, 1-convex;
- the intersection of 1-visible compact bodies is a 1-visible body.

We shall describe some illustrative examples in the space $\mathbb{R}^3$.

a. Let $W = I^3 \setminus V$, where I^3 is the cube $-1 \leq x, y, z \leq +1$ and V is the vertical cylinder $x^2 + y^2 < 0.01$. It is obvious that any point $M \notin W$ is contained in some straight line disjoint from W.

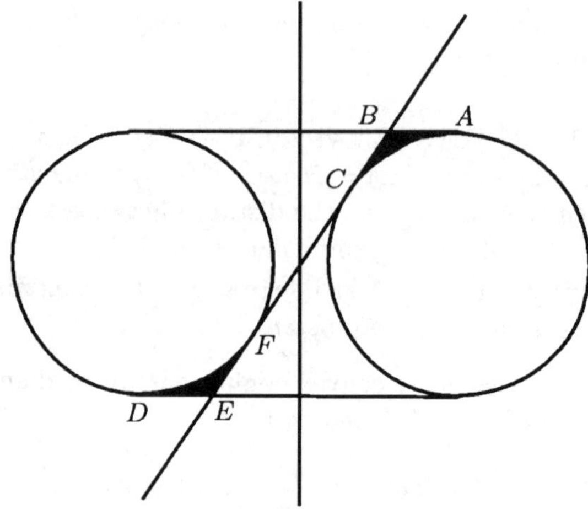

Figure 1.1: The points in the black triangles ABC and DEF cannot be seen on any projection of the torus

b. If two 1-visible bodies in $\mathbb{R}^3$ have homeomorphic projections onto any plane, it is not true that they are homeomorphic themselves. If I^3 and V are as in the previous example, $W = I^3 \setminus V$, V_1 and V_2 are the cylinders $x^2+z^2 < 0.01$ and $(x-0.5)^2+z^2 < 0.01$, respectively, then the 1-visible body $W_1 = I^3 \setminus (V \cup V_1)$ is not homeomorphic to $W_2 = I^3 \setminus (V \cup V_2)$, since $V \cap V_2$ is empty and $V \cap V_1$ is not. However, it is easy to see that the projections of these bodies W_1 and W_2 onto any plane are pairwise homeomorphic.

c. The standard smooth torus of revolution in $\mathbb{R}^3$:

$$(x^2 + y^2 + z^2 + 24)^2 = 100(x^2 + y^2)$$

is not a 1-visible body since in its "hole" there are some points close to the lines $z = \pm 1$ which cannot be seen on any projection of this torus (see Figure 1.1).

d. A. V. Kuz'minyh has constructed a smooth embedding of the 2-dimensional torus into $\mathbb{R}^3$ that gives a 1-visible body: consider the cube I^3 with the vertices $ABCDA'B'C'D'$ and compose the closed polygon $ABB'C'D'DA$. Let us smooth the angles of this polygon and consider

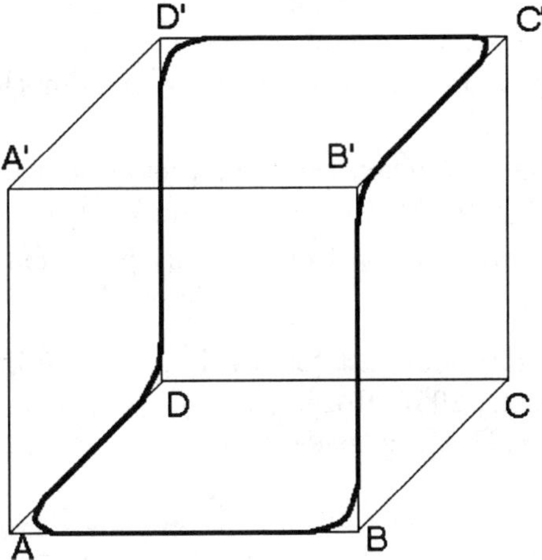

Figure 1.2: A smooth embedding of a thin torus into three-dimensional space

a small tubular neighborhood of this smooth closed line (see Figure 1.2). The closure of this neighborhood is 1-visible.

e. One can construct a 2-convex compact body that is not 2-visible:

Consider a compact body $W = I^4 \setminus (A_x \cup A_y \cup A_z) \subset \mathbb{R}^4$, where I^4 is the four-dimensional cube $-1 \leq x, y, z, t \leq +1$ and the open sets A_x, A_y, A_z are defined by

$$A_x = \{-0.1 < |x| < +0.1;\ 0.0 \leq t < 0.4\},$$
$$A_y = \{-0.1 < |y| < +0.1;\ 0.3 < t < 0.7\},$$
$$A_z = \{-0.1 < |z| < +0.1;\ 0.6 < t \leq 1.0\}.$$

Clearly, the axis Ot is disjoint from this compact body W; on the other hand, it is not difficult to verify that

(i) the axis Ot is not contained in any two-dimensional plane disjoint from W; hence, this body W is not 2-visible in $\mathbb{R}^4$;

(ii) any point in any of the sets $A_x \cap I^4$, $A_y \cap I^4$ and $A_z \cap I^4$ is contained in some two-dimensional plane disjoint from W: for the points of $A_x \cap I^4$, this plane is parallel to the coordinate plane Oyz; for the points of $A_y \cap I^4$, this plane is parallel to Oxz, etc.

Thus, the compact body W is 2-convex in $\mathbb{R}^4$.

Definition 1.1.6. Two compact sets in a vector space will be called *parallel* or *directly homothetic* if one of them can be obtained from the other by a parallel translation or, respectively, by a homothety with a suitable center.

In the particular case when the homothety coefficient equals -1, these two sets are called *centrally symmetric to each other.*

We shall call a compact set A in a vector space *centrally symmetric* if A is parallel to $-A$.

We use these definitions just for brevity, because in the literature (see, for example, Groemer, 1987; Rogers, 1965), the above defined parallel sets are often called *translation equivalent*, etc.

Definition 1.1.7. Given two sets A_1 and A_2 in a vector space $\mathbf{E}$ and a group $G \subseteq GL(\mathbf{E})$ of linear transformations of $\mathbf{E}$, we shall call these sets *G-congruent* if for some element $g \in G$ the sets $g(A_2)$ and A_1 are parallel in $\mathbf{E}$.

Usually, we shall consider the case of the special orthogonal groups $SO(k)$ and all the isometries of the Euclidean spaces will be assumed to be orientation preserving.

Definition 1.1.8. Let V be a subset of a vector space $\mathbf{E}$ and let G be a subgroup of the group of the linear transformations of this space. We shall say that the set V *has no G-symmetries* if for any non-identity element $g \in G$ the sets V and $g(V)$ are not parallel in $\mathbf{E}$.

Definition 1.1.9. Two sets in a Euclidean space will be called *similar* (or *SO-similar*) if they are equivalent with respect to the composition of an (orientation preserving) isometry and a homothety.

Petty and McKinney (1987) constructed surprising examples of pairs of centrally symmetric bodies of revolution in $\mathbb{R}^n$ whose projections onto any two-dimensional plane are $SO(2)$-similar and have symmetries with respect to the antipodal involution. Gardner and Volčič (1994) showed that very often the convex bodies in these pairs are not affinely equivalent. So, for some transformation groups our Main Question has in general an unexpected answer (see Section 3.1).

Since the order of stability in reconstruction of a body from its projections depends on the metric used in the class of the objects under consideration, we shall list some of these metrics:

Definition 1.1.10. *The Hausdorff distance* between compact sets in a Euclidean space is

$$\rho_h(M,N) = \max\{\sup_{x\in M}\inf_{y\in N}|x-y|,\ \sup_{y\in N}\inf_{x\in M}|x-y|\}.$$

Definition 1.1.11. *Translative distance* between compact sets in a Euclidean space $\mathbf{E}^n$ is

$$\rho_t(M,N) = \inf_{p\in\mathbf{E}^n}\rho_h(M,N+p).$$

This translative distance was used by Groemer (1987).

Stability theorem: *Let $M, N \subset \mathbb{R}^n$, $n \geq 3$, be two convex compact bodies and $\varepsilon \geq 0$. If for any $\omega \in S^{n-1}$ the projections $M(\omega)$, $N(\omega)$ are parallel to within the Hausdorff distance ε: $\rho_t(M(\omega),N(\omega)) < \varepsilon$, then $\rho_t(M,N) < (1+2\sqrt{2})\varepsilon$.*

Groemer notes that the coefficient $(1+2\sqrt{2})$ in this inequality does not seem to be the best possible and we have no better estimate at our disposal as well.

Definition 1.1.12. For any group G of transformations of the Euclidean space $\mathbb{R}^n$ one can define the following distance between compact sets in this space:

$$\rho_G(M,N) = \inf_{g\in G}\rho_h(M,g(N)).$$

Helmut Groemer studied the stability of recovering the shapes of convex bodies in the case of positively homothetic transformations of projections of these convex bodies (see Groemer, 1987, 1994). We shall study the corresponding stability problems for the group SI of all orientation preserving isometries of the space.

Definition 1.1.13. For a nonempty set $V \subset \mathbf{E}^n$ in a Euclidean space $\mathbf{E}^n$ we shall call the set

$$V^* = \{x \in \mathbf{E}^n \mid \langle x,y\rangle \leq 1 \text{ for all } y \in V\}$$

the polar set of V (see, for example, Gardner, 1995). It can be easily verified that for a given hyperplane $P(\omega) \subset \mathbb{R}^n$ and a convex body $V \subset \mathbb{R}^n$ one has $V^* \cap P(\omega) = (V(\omega))^*$. Similar identity holds for the subspaces of higher codimension as well. Therefore, most of the results concerning projections of the convex compact bodies can be formulated for the sections of these bodies and vice versa using this operation of *polar duality*.

1.2. TRANSLATION EQUIVALENCE OF PROJECTIONS. PRELIMINARY RESULTS

The Main Question (**MQ**) in the case of parallel translation of projections has been studied thoroughly in literature from different viewpoints (Süss, 1932; Aleksandrov, 1937; Groemer, 1986; etc.) since parallel convex bodies have the same width and brightness functions, mixed volumes and other useful numerical geometric characteristics.

In particular, Süss proved that if the projections of two convex compact bodies $V_1, V_2 \subset \mathbb{R}^n$, $n > 2$, onto any hyperplane are parallel in this hyperplane, then these bodies are parallel in the ambient space $\mathbb{R}^n$ themselves. Groemer has obtained stability estimates for this uniqueness up to a parallel translation.

We shall generalize this result in several directions considering wider transformation groups, wider classes of multidimensional objects in a Euclidean space, etc.

In practical reconstruction problems, especially in tomographic investigations, sometimes it happens that full information on the projections of a multidimensional object is not available. So, in this section we shall relax the condition in Süss's lemma that all projections of two convex compact bodies are parallel in the corresponding hyperplanes.

Similar problems of optimization of the projection data have been studied in many publications on geometry and mathematical tomography (Kirillov, 1961; Gel'fand and Graev, 1968; Tuy, 1983; Finch, 1985; Ayupova and Golubyatnikov, 1990; Groemer, 1994; etc.), for example, Groemer considered the so-called *full* collection of hyperplanes in a Euclidean space, which is sufficient for the stable reconstruction of shapes of compact convex bodies.

Lemma 1.2.1. *Let $\Omega_1 \subset S^{n-1}$ be a set of unit vectors that has nonempty intersection with any great $(n-2)$-dimensional sphere. If the projections of convex compact sets $V_1, V_2 \subset \mathbb{R}^n$ onto any hyperplane $P(\omega)$ for $\omega \in \Omega_1$ coincide: $V_1(\omega) = V_2(\omega)$, then these convex compact sets V_1 and V_2 coincide themselves.*

The proof is almost obvious. Note that the same result holds in the complex Euclidean space $\mathbb{C}^n$, where the set Ω_1 should be taken in the unit sphere $S^{2n-1} \subset \mathbb{C}^n$. We mention this result here just for the completeness of exposition because these propositions (the real and the complex one) correspond to the identical transformations of the projections of the bodies in the sense of our main question **MQ**.

Lemma 1.2.2. *If $\omega_1, \omega_2, \omega_3 \subset S^{n-1}$ are noncoplanar unit vectors in a Euclidean space $\mathbf{E}^n$ and the projections of convex compact bodies V_1 and V_2 onto the planes $P(\omega_1)$ and $P(\omega_2)$ coincide and the projections $V_1(\omega_3)$ and $V_2(\omega_3)$ are parallel in the plane $P(\omega_3)$, then $V_1(\omega_3) = V_2(\omega_3)$.*

Proof. Let $P_{i,j} = P(\omega_i) \cap P(\omega_j)$, $i, j = 1, 2, 3$, be the intersections of the hyperplanes orthogonal to the vectors ω_k, $k = 1, 2, 3$. Consider the projections of V_1 and V_2 onto the $(n-2)$-dimensional planes $P_{1,3}$ and $P_{2,3}$ which lie in the hyperplane $P(\omega_3)$; these projections coincide because the procedure of projection onto $P_{1,3}$ can be done in two steps: first, one projects onto $P(\omega_1)$, where the projections of V_1 and V_2 coincide by hypothesis, and then onto $P_{1,3}$, where the projections of V_1 and V_2 coincide again. Similarly, it can be established that the projections of these bodies onto $P_{2,3}$ coincide as well.

Suppose that the projection $V_1(\omega_3)$ can be obtained from $V_2(\omega_3)$ by a parallel translation by a nonzero vector a. The projection of this vector a onto the plane $P_{1,3}$ is equal to zero because the projections of V_1 and V_2 onto $P_{1,3}$ coincide. Similarly, the projection of a onto the plane $P_{2,3}$ is equal to zero as well. Since the linear span of $P_{1,3} \cup P_{2,3}$ coincides with the hyperplane $P(\omega_3)$, one has $a = 0$ and hence $V_1(\omega_3) = V_2(\omega_3)$. □

Theorem 1.2.1. *If the set $\Omega_2 \subset S^{n-1}$ contains three noncoplanar vectors and intersects every great $(n-2)$-dimensional sphere, and for any $\omega \in \Omega_2$ the projections $V_1(\omega)$ and $V_2(\omega)$ of convex compact bodies $V_1, V_2 \subset \mathbb{R}^n$ onto the hyperplane $P(\omega)$ are parallel, then these bodies V_1 and V_2 are parallel in $\mathbb{R}^n$ themselves.*

Proof. Given three noncoplanar vectors $\omega_1, \omega_2, \omega_3 \subset \Omega_2$, consider the convex body V_1', obtained from V_1 by a parallel translation such that the projections of V_2 and V_1' onto the plane $P(\omega_1)$ coincide. The projection of V_2 onto the hyperplane $P(\omega_2)$ can be obtained from the corresponding projection of V_1' by a parallel translation by a vector b orthogonal to the plane $P(\omega_1) \cap P(\omega_2)$ as was shown in Lemma 1.2.2. Let us translate the body V_1' in the direction of ω_1 so that for the obtained body V_1'' the projections $V_1''(\omega_2)$ and $V_2(\omega_2)$ coincide. Let α be the angle between the vectors ω_1 and ω_2. The length of the translation V_1' to V_1'' is equal to $|b| \cdot (\sin \alpha)^{-1}$. As was shown above, the projections of V_1'' and V_2 onto the plane $P(\omega_3)$ also coincide. If $\omega \in \Omega_2$, then at least one of the triples $\{\omega, \omega_2, \omega_3\}$, $\{\omega, \omega_3, \omega_1\}$, $\{\omega, \omega_1, \omega_2\}$ is linearly independent. Hence, the projections of V_1'' and V_2 onto $P(\omega_3)$ also coincide, and our theorem follows from Lemma 1.2.1. □

It is not difficult to verify that this theorem holds for the sets $\Omega_2 \subset S^{n-1}$ whose closures intersect every great $(n-2)$-dimensional sphere.

The condition of linear independence of the vectors $\omega_1, \omega_2, \omega_3 \in \Omega_2$ is essential: let $\Omega_2 \subset S^2$ be an equator $E(\omega)$. Consider all the figures of constant width w in the plane $P(\omega)$ of this equator. The projections of all the cylinders of height h over all these figures onto the vertical planes that are perpendicular to $P(\omega)$ are the rectangles with base w and height h, so they are parallel, but one cannot make all the projections of these *a priori* noncongruent cylinders onto all the planes orthogonal to the vectors $\omega_* \in \Omega_2$ coincide at once.

In the same way one can prove the complex analogue of Theorem 1.2.1:

Theorem 1.2.2. *If $\Omega_2 \subset S^{2n-1} \subset \mathbb{C}^n$, $n > 2$, contains three noncoplanar vectors and intersects every great $(2n-2)$-dimensional sphere and for any $\omega \in \Omega_2$ the projections $V_1(\omega)$ and $V_2(\omega)$ of convex compact bodies V_1 and V_2 in $\mathbb{C}^n$ onto the hyperplane $P(\omega)$ are parallel, then the bodies V_1 and V_2 are parallel in $\mathbb{C}^n$ themselves.*

Following the idea of our Main Question **MQ**, we shall consider wider group of transformations of projections.

Lemma 1.2.3. *Let $V_1, V_2 \subset \mathbb{R}^n$, $n > 2$, be compact convex bodies and let $\Omega_2 \subset S^{n-1}$ be the same as in Theorem 1.2.1 and let the projections $V_1(\omega)$ and $V_2(\omega)$ be homothetic to each other for all $\omega \in \Omega_2$ (the homothety coefficient λ is not assumed to be constant, independent of the direction ω). Then V_1 and V_2 are directly homothetic in $\mathbb{R}^n$.*

Lemma 1.2.4. *Let $V_1, V_2 \subset \mathbb{C}^n$, $n > 2$, be compact convex bodies and let $\Omega_2 \subset S^{2n-1}$ be the same as in Theorem 1.2.2 and let the projections $V_1(\omega)$ and $V_2(\omega)$ be homothetic to each other for all $\omega \in \Omega_2$. If their projections onto any $(n-2)$-dimensional complex subspace P^{n-2} have no $U(1)$-symmetries (as in the previous lemma, the homothety coefficient $\lambda(\omega)$ is not assumed to be constant, independent of the direction ω), then V_1 and V_2 are directly homothetic in $\mathbb{C}^n$.*

Proof. In the real case, Lemma 1.2.3 was proved by Hadwiger (1963), (see also Rogers, 1965). We shall give the proof of the complex variant of this lemma.

First, note that the homothety coefficient $\lambda = \lambda(P(\omega)) = \lambda(\omega)$ actually does not depend on the direction ω of the projection. In fact, let the unit vectors ω_1 and ω_2 be nonparallel in $\mathbb{C}^n$ and let $\lambda(\omega_1) \neq \lambda(\omega_2)$. We shall denote by $P^{n-2}(\omega_1, \omega_2)$ the intersection $P(\omega_1) \cap P(\omega_2)$. It is not difficult to verify that the projections $V_1(P^{n-2}(\omega_1, \omega_2))$ and $V_2(P^{n-2}(\omega_1, \omega_2))$ of the bodies V_1 and V_2 onto this intersection are homothetic to each other with homothety coefficient $\lambda(\omega_1)$ and, at the same time, with coefficient $\lambda(\omega_2)$. The coincidence of the absolute values $|\lambda(\omega_1)| = |\lambda(\omega_2)|$ follows from the compactness of the bodies V_1 and V_2. The absence of $U(1)$-symmetries of the projections $V_1(P^{n-2}(\omega_1, \omega_2))$ and $V_2(P^{n-2}(\omega_1, \omega_2))$ implies the coincidence of the arguments of these homothety coefficients.

Since the independence of this coefficient on ω is established, the proof of this lemma follows from Theorem 1.2.2. □

All these results, which we have obtained for the convex bodies in the Euclidean spaces, can be formulated for $(n-k)$-convex bodies as well:

Lemma 1.2.5. *Let W_1, W_2 be compact $(n-k)$-convex bodies in a Euclidean space $\mathbf{E}^n$, $n > 2$, $k > 1$. If their projections $W_1(P^k)$ and $W_2(P^k)$ onto any k-dimensional plane $P^k \subset \mathbf{E}^n$ coincide, then these bodies W_1 and W_2 coincide in $\mathbf{E}^n$ themselves.*

Proof. Suppose that some point $x \in W_1$ is not contained in the $(n-k)$-convex body W_2. Then there is an $(n-k)$-dimensional plane $P^{n-k} \subset \mathbf{E}^n$ which contains x and is disjoint from W_1. Let $P^{\perp}$ be the orthogonal complement of P^{n-k}. It is obvious that the projection of W_1 onto $P^{\perp}$ does not coincide with the corresponding projection of W_2, since the projection of the point $x \in W_1$ in the "direction" of the plane P^{n-k} is contained in the projection of W_1 and is not contained in the projection of W_2. □

Lemma 1.2.6. *Let W_1 and W_2 be compact $(n-k)$-convex bodies in a Euclidean space $\mathbf{E}^n$, $n > 2$, $k > 1$. If their projections $W_1(P^k)$ and $W_2(P^k)$ onto any k-dimensional plane in $\mathbf{E}^n$ are parallel, then these bodies W_1 and W_2 are parallel in $\mathbf{E}^n$ themselves.*

Proof. Since the projection of a convex hull is the convex hull of the projection, it is easy to see that the projections of the convex hulls $\operatorname{conv} W_1$ and $\operatorname{conv} W_2$ of the bodies W_1 and W_2 onto any k-dimensional plane are parallel. It follows from Süss's lemma, that $\operatorname{conv} W_1$ and $\operatorname{conv} W_2$ are parallel. Let T be the corresponding parallel translation: $T(\operatorname{conv} W_1) = \operatorname{conv} W_2$. Hence, the projections of $T(\operatorname{conv} W_1)$ and $\operatorname{conv} W_2$ onto any k-dimensional plane coincide, and it is obvious that the projections of $T(W_1)$ and W_2 onto any k-dimensional plane coincide as well. Thus, the equality $T(W_1) = W_2$ follows from Lemma 1.2.6. □

Clearly, these two lemmas are valid in the real, complex and quaternionic finite-dimensional Euclidean spaces. They can be generalized to the case of homothetic projections of the $(n-k)$-convex bodies in n-dimensional Euclidean space. For example, the following lemma can be easily deduced from the previous results of this section.

Lemma 1.2.7. *Let W_1, W_2 be compact $(n-k)$-convex bodies in a Euclidean space $\mathbf{E}^n$, $n > 2$, $k > 1$. If their projections $W_1(P^k)$ and $W_2(P^k)$ onto any k-dimensional plane in $\mathbf{E}^n$ are homothetic (as above, the homothety coefficient is not assumed to be constant), then these bodies W_1 and W_2 are directly homothetic in $\mathbf{E}^n$ themselves.*

The analogues of all these results hold in infinite-dimensional spaces as well.

Lemma 1.2.8. *Let V_1 and V_2 be convex compact sets in a separable Hilbert space $\mathcal{H}$ and let their orthogonal projections onto any k-dimensional subspace be parallel in this subspace, $2 \leq k < \infty$. Then V_1 and V_2 are parallel in $\mathcal{H}$.*

This lemma easily follows from the considerations of the finite ε-nets of the compact sets V_1 and V_2 for sufficiently small ε.

The following statements can be obtained in a similar way, see Anikonov *et al.* (1997) and Golubyatnikov (1982b).

Lemma 1.2.9. *An analytic, compact, connected, closed k-dimesional manifold analytically imbedded in $\mathbb{R}^n$, $n \geq 3$, $n > k \geq 1$, is uniquely determined by its convex hull.*

Theorem 1.2.3. *If the projections of two compact, analytic, connected and closed hypersurfaces $M_1, M_2 \subset \mathbb{R}^n$, $n \geq 3$, onto any hyperplane are parallel, then these hypersurfaces are parallel themselves.*

Chapter 2.

$SO(2)$-congruence of projections

2.1. THE CASE OF CONVEX BODIES

Now, we shall generalize Süss's lemma for another class of transformations of projections of convex bodies, which is wider than that of parallel translations and more complicated than those of homotheties. Most of the statements presented here were obtained in Golubyatnikov (1988, 1990, 1991, 1995b).

The main result of this section is the following theorem.

Theorem 2.1.1. *If V_1 and V_2 are compact convex bodies in $\mathbb{R}^3$ such that for any unit vector ω their projections $V_1(\omega)$ and $V_2(\omega)$ onto the plane $P(\omega)$ are $SO(2)$-congruent and have no $SO(2)$-symmetries, then V_1 and V_2 are either parallel or centrally symmetric to each other in $\mathbb{R}^3$.*

Proof. For a fixed orientation in $\mathbb{R}^3$, let us denote by $\varphi(\omega)$ the least angle φ in the absolute value such that the projection $V_1(\omega)$ is obtained from $V_2(\omega)$ by the rotation through the angle φ with a suitable center of rotation. If these projections are parallel, we set $\varphi(\omega) = 0$. For purely geometrical reasons, the rotations through the angles π and $-\pi$ are identified with each other. It is not difficult to verify that the above defined *rotation function* $\varphi : S^2 \longrightarrow S^1$ satisfies the following identity:

$$\varphi(\omega) = -\varphi(-\omega).$$

This equation plays the central role in the proof of our theorem. Here the signs of the angles are determined by the unit normals $\omega \perp P(\omega)$ and

$-\omega \perp P(-\omega)$. We shall denote by $E(\omega)$ the great circle (equator) $E(\omega) = S^2 \cap P(\omega)$.

Clearly, if the projections of the convex bodies V_1 and V_2 in $\mathbb{R}^3$ onto any plane $P(\omega)$ are congruent, then the perimeters $L_1(\omega)$ and $L_2(\omega)$ and the areas $S_1(\omega)$ and $S_2(\omega)$ of these projections are equal even in the case of $O(2)$-congruence. That is why the authors of the articles devoted to the numerical characteristics of projections and sections of (convex) bodies usually do not need to distinguish between the orientable and nonorientable cases (see, for example, Pogorelov, 1973; Kuz'minykh, 1973; Ball, 1991; Montejano, 1991a; etc.).

These perimeters $L_1(\omega)$ and $L_2(\omega)$ can be expressed in terms of the width functions w_i and the support functions H_i of these convex bodies $w_1(\omega) = H_1(\omega) + H_1(-\omega)$ and $w_2(\omega) = H_2(\omega) + H_2(-\omega)$ with the help of the spherical Radon transform:

$$L_1(\omega) = L_2(\omega) = \frac{1}{2} \int\limits_{E(\omega)} w_1(s)\, \mathrm{d}s = \frac{1}{2} \int\limits_{E(\omega)} w_2(s)\, \mathrm{d}s. \tag{2.1.1}$$

A similar expression can be derived for the area functions $S_i(\omega)$, $i = 1, 2$. As was shown in Blaschke (1949), each of these integral equations has a unique solution. Thus, the convex bodies V_1 and V_2 have the same width in any direction.

It follows immediately from this fact that if two centrally symmetric convex bodies have the same width function, then they are parallel to each other (see, for example, Aleksandrov, 1937; Schneider, 1970). Thus, the main difficulty in our theorem is connected with the asymmetric case.

A. V. Kuz'minyh studied the problem of congruence of convex bodies with $SO(2)$-congruent asymmetric projections under the following condition: these bodies should have finitely many diameters. It is obvious that the class of convex bodies satisfying this restriction constitutes an open everywhere dense set with respect to the Hausdorff metric in the class of all compact convex bodies in a Euclidean space. To the best of the author's knowledge, these results have not been published. We shall use this approach later in Section 3.2, where our Main Question is considered in the case of $SO(3)$-congruent projections of convex bodies onto 3-dimensional planes in $\mathbb{R}^n$, $n \geq 4$.

Lemma 2.1.1. *If for all unit vectors $\omega \in S^2$ the projections $V_1(\omega)$ and $V_2(\omega)$ have no $SO(2)$-symmetries, then $\varphi : S^2 \longrightarrow S^1$ is a continuous function of the direction of the projection ω.*

Proof. If $\lim_{i\to\infty}(\omega_i) = \omega_0$ on the sphere and $\lim_{t\to\infty}\varphi(\omega_i) \neq \varphi(\omega_0)$, then we can find a subsequence $\{\psi_j\} \subset \{\omega_i\}$ on the compact space S^2 such that $\lim_{j\to\infty}\varphi(\psi_j) = \varphi_1 \neq \varphi(\omega_0)$. It is easy to verify that the projections $V_1(\omega_0)$ and $V_2(\omega_0)$ are $SO(2)$-congruent with respect to rotations through the angle $\varphi(\omega_0)$ and through the angle φ_1, which is impossible because of the absence of the $SO(2)$-symmetries of these projections. □

Clearly, if for some $\omega \in S^2$ the projections $V_1(\omega)$ and $V_2(\omega)$ have $SO(2)$-symmetries, then the rotation mapping φ cannot be defined correctly.

If $\varphi(\omega) \equiv 0$ on the sphere S^2, then $V_1(\omega)$ and $V_2(\omega)$ are parallel, and our theorem follows from Süss's lemma.

If $\varphi(\omega) \equiv \pi$ for all $\omega \in S^2$, we consider a convex body V_1' obtained by a certain central symmetry of V_1. It is obvious that for any $\omega \in S^2$ the projections $V_1'(\omega)$ and $V_2(\omega)$ are parallel in the plane $P(\omega)$, and it follows from Süss's lemma that V_1' and V_2 are parallel in $\mathbb{R}^3$. Hence, in this case V_1 and V_2 are centrally symmetric to each other with respect to some center.

Now, suppose that there is a vector $\omega_0 \in S^2$ such that $\pi > \varphi(\omega_0) > 0$. Consider all meridians $m(t)$ on S^2 that join the points ω_0 and $-\omega_0$, where $0 \leq t \leq 2\pi$ and t parametrizes the points on the great circle $C(\omega_0)$. For the continuous mapping $\varphi : S^2 \longrightarrow S^1$ we shall denote by $\varphi^{-1}(0)$ and by $\varphi^{-1}(\pi)$, respectively, the preimages of the points $0, \pi \in S^1$. Let $[\varphi^{-1}(0)]$ and $[\varphi^{-1}(\pi)]$ be the sets of nonisolated points of these preimages and let $\Sigma \subset S^2$ be the set of all the unit vectors ω such that the projections $V_1(\omega)$ and $V_2(\omega)$ have constant width. The value of this width does not depend on the choice of $\omega \in \Sigma$ because any two great circles on the sphere S^2 intersect. It is easy to see that all the sets $[\varphi^{-1}(0)]$, $[\varphi^{-1}(\pi)]$, $\varphi^{-1}(0)$, $\varphi^{-1}(\pi)$ and Σ are closed and centrally symmetric on S^2 with respect to the antipodal mapping.

For any angle $\alpha \in S^1$, the closed set $\varphi^{-1}(\alpha)$ can be defined exactly in the same way.

Lemma 2.1.2. *For the continuous mapping φ, one of the sets $\varphi^{-1}(0)$ and $\varphi^{-1}(\pi)$ intersects all the meridians $m(t)$.*

Proof. The zero meridian $m(0)$ determines a continuous mapping of triples of the spaces:

$$\mu_0 : ([-\pi/2, \pi/2], -\pi/2, \pi/2) \longrightarrow (S^1, -\varphi(\omega_0), \varphi(\omega_0)).$$

The corresponding homomorphism of the integer homology groups

$$Z \approx H_1([-\pi/2, \pi/2], -\pi/2, \pi/2) \\ \longrightarrow H_1(S^1, \varphi^{-1}(-\omega_0), \varphi^{-1}(\omega_0)) \approx Z \oplus Z$$

maps the generator of the group Z to the element $(n_1, n_2) \in Z \oplus Z$ such that $n_1 + n_2$ is an odd number, because the angles $\varphi(-\omega_0)$ and $\varphi(\omega_0)$ lie in different half-planes with respect to the horizontal line containing 0 and π, and the intersection index of $\mu_0(m(0))$ and this horizontal line is equal to 1. The coefficient n_1 corresponds to the left arc $\{\varphi(-\omega_0), \varphi(\omega_0)\}$ of the circle S^1, and n_2 corresponds to the right one. As t varies from 0 to $\pi/2$, we obtain a homotopy μ_t of the mapping μ_0; hence, the element (n_1, n_2) does not depend on t. If n_1 is odd, then the left arc $\{\varphi(-\omega_0), \varphi(\omega_0)\}$, which contains π, is covered under a mapping of all the meridians $m(t)$. If n_2 is odd, then the right arc $\{\varphi(-\omega_0), \varphi(\omega_0)\}$, which contains 0, is covered under a mapping of all meridians. □

Corollary 2.1.1. Under the assumptions of Lemma 2.1.2, one of the sets $[\varphi^{-1}(0)]$ and $[\varphi^{-1}(\pi)]$ intersects all meridians $m(t)$.

As above, if all the meridians $m(t)$ intersect the preimage $\varphi^{-1}(\pi)$, we replace the body V_1 by V_1', which is obtained by the central symmetry, in order to change the roles of the preimages $\varphi^{-1}(0)$ and $\varphi^{-1}(\pi)$. For the convex bodies V_1' and V_2, all the meridians $m(t)$ intersect the preimage $\varphi^{-1}(0)$. Thus, we may assume in the sequel that such a change has been made if necessary.

Lemma 2.1.3. *If $[\varphi^{-1}(0)]$ is not a great circle on S^2 and intersects all the meridians $m(t)$, then there are two nonparallel vectors $\omega_1, \omega_2 \in [\varphi^{-1}(0)]$ such that for a dense set of parameters t in $E(\omega_0)$ the corresponding meridians $m(t)$ intersect the set $[\varphi^{-1}(0)]$ at points which are not coplanar with ω_1 and ω_2.*

Proof. If there are two different points of $[\varphi^{-1}(0)]$ on some meridian $m(t_1)$, we take these two points for the required ω_1 and ω_2. All the meridians except $m(t_1)$ and its antipodal meridian intersect $[\varphi^{-1}(0)]$ at some point that is not coplanar with these two vectors.

If there is exactly one point of $[\varphi^{-1}(0)]$ on every $m(t)$, we shall denote it by $\omega(t)$; note that in this case $[\varphi^{-1}(0)]$ is homeomorphic to a circle. For every $\omega_1 \in [\varphi^{-1}(0)]$, consider the family of all great circles $E(\omega_1, t)$ containing ω_1 and $\omega(t) \neq \omega_1$. By the assumptions, $[\varphi^{-1}(0)]$ is not contained in any great circle on S^2. On the other hand, it is impossible to place a continuum of nonintersecting intervals on a circle; hence, the intersection of at least one of these circles $E(\omega_1, t_1)$ with $[\varphi^{-1}(0)]$ has dense complement in $[\varphi^{-1}(0)]$. We take the vector $\omega(t_1)$ corresponding to this circle for the required vector ω_2. □

For the vectors $\omega_1, \omega_2 \in [\varphi^{-1}(0)]$ obtained in this lemma, we perform a parallel translation of V_1 (or V_1', in the case when all the meridians $m(t)$ intersect the set $[\varphi^{-1}(\pi)]$) so that the projections of the obtained body V_1'' onto the planes $P(\omega_1)$ and $P(\omega_2)$ coincide with the corresponding projections of the body V_2.

Take any t^* which belongs to the dense subset of $E(\omega_1)$ defined in Lemma 2.1.3 so that $\omega(t^*) \in [\varphi^{-1}(0)]$ is not coplanar with ω_1 and ω_2. It follows from Lemma 1.2.2 that the projections $V_1''(\omega(t^*))$ coincide with $V_2(\omega(t^*))$ for any t^* that belongs to such a dense subset. The support functions $H_2(\omega)$ and $H_1''(\omega)$ of the convex bodies V_2 and V_1'' coincide on all the great circles $E(\omega(t^*)) \subset S^2$. The intersection of the union of these circles with the equator $E(\omega_0)$ is a dense set on this equator; hence, the continuous functions $H_2(\omega)$ and $H_1''(\omega)$ coincide on this equator. This contradicts to the assumption $\pi > \varphi(\omega_0) > 0$.

So, we have proved Theorem 2.1.1 for $n = 3$ in the case when the preimage $[\varphi^{-1}(0)]$ (or $[\varphi^{-1}(\pi)]$) is not contained in any great circle of the unit sphere S^2.

Lemma 2.1.4. *If the projections of the convex bodies V_1 and V_2 in $\mathbb{R}^3$ onto any plane are $SO(2)$-congruent, then $S^2 = \varphi^{-1}(0) \cup \varphi^{-1}(\pi) \cup \Sigma$.*

Proof. Note that in this lemma we do not assume that the projections have no $SO(2)$-symmetries. We denote by $\{\varphi(\omega)\}$ the set of all the angles $\varphi(\omega) \in S^1$ such that the projection $V_1(\omega)$ transforms to the projection $V_2(\omega)$ by a rotation through the angle $\varphi(\omega)$.

If the open set $F = S^2 \setminus (\varphi^{-1}(0) \cup \varphi^{-1}(\pi) \cup \Sigma)$ is not empty, consider any $\omega_1 \in F$. If the set $\{\varphi(\omega_1)\}$ contains the angle πa for an irrational a, then the angles $\pi a k$, where k are integer, form a dense set in the circle $E(\omega_1)$. Therefore, the widths of the bodies V_1 and V_2 coincide on this circle, which contradicts the choice of ω_1.

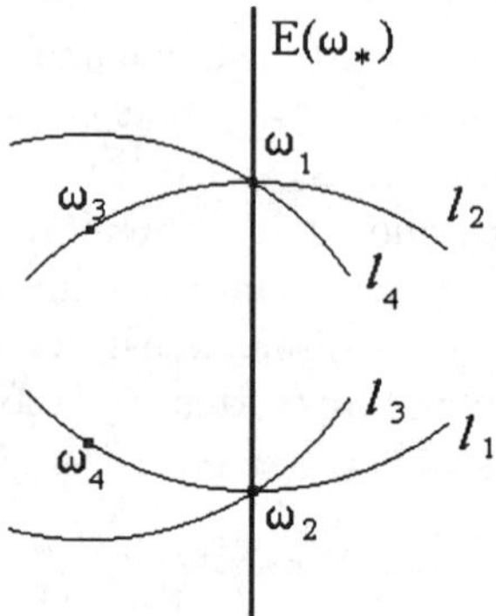

Figure 2.1: The arcs l_1, l_2, l_3, and l_4.

Hence, if the set F is not empty, then it is a finite or countable union of the sets $F(p/q)$ composed of vectors ω such that $\pi p/q \in \{\varphi(\omega)\}$ for coprime integers p and q.

It follows from the Baire category theorem that at least one of these sets $F(p/q)$ is dense in an open domain $D \subset S^2$. The rest of the proof of Lemma 2.1.4 is based on the following lemma.

Lemma 2.1.5. *If V_1, V_2 and D are as above, p and q are positive coprime integers, $p < q$ and for any $\omega \in D$ one has $\pi p/q \in \{\varphi(\omega)\}$, then for these vectors $\omega \in D$ the projections $V_1(\omega)$ and $V_2(\omega)$ have constant width.*

Proof of Lemma 2.1.5. If the assertion of this lemma is false, then there exists some $\omega_* \in D$ such that for a certain vector $\omega_1 \in E(\omega_*)$ the width $w_1(\omega_1) = M$ of the body V_1 is maximal on the great circle $E(\omega_*)$ and is not constant in any neighborhood of ω_1 in this circle. Let ω_2 be the unit vector in $E(\omega_*)$ that is obtained by rotation of ω_1 through the angle $\varphi(\omega_*)$ with the direction of rotations determined by the normal vector ω_*. Also, let $S(\omega_1, p/q) \subset S^2$ be the circle with center ω_1 and radius $\pi p/q$ in the standard metric of the unit sphere. Since D is open, there is an open arc l_1 on this circle such that $\omega_2 \in l_1$ and the widths of V_1 and V_2 in the directions of the vectors corresponding to l_1 are equal to $M = w_1(\omega_2) = w_2(\omega_2)$.

Similarly, on the circle $S(\omega_2, p/q) \subset S^2$ with the same radius and center at ω_2 there is an open arc l_2 containing ω_1 and such that the widths of V_1 and V_2 in the directions of the vectors corresponding to l_2 are also equal to M.

Take any point $\omega_4 \in l_1$ such that $\omega_4 \neq \omega_2$ and consider an arc l_4 on the circle $S(\omega_4, p/q)$ such that $\omega_2 \in l_4$ and the widths of V_1 and V_2 in the directions corresponding to l_3 are equal to M as well. In the same manner, we construct an arc $l_3 \subset S(\omega_3, p/q)$ with center $\omega_3 \in l_2$ such that $\omega_3 \neq \omega_2$ (see Figure 2.1). Let ω_c be a vector in a small neighborhood of $\omega_1 \in E(\omega_*)$ such that $w_1(\omega_c) = w_2(\omega_c) = c \neq M$. From the construction of these figures "X", $X = l_1 \cup l_3$ or $X = l_2 \cup l_4$, which depend on the vectors ω, we see that on different figures X's corresponding to different values of c the widths of the bodies V_1 and V_2 are constant, hence the different figures "X" are mutually disjoint. The cardinality of the set of these c is that of continuum but it is well known that the cardinality of a set of mutually disjoint figures "X" on the plane or on the sphere S^2 is strictly less than continuum. Therefore, in some neighborhood of ω_1 in $E(\omega_*)$ the width function w_1 must be constant, which contradicts the choice of the vector ω_1. Hence, the width functions w_1 and w_2 are constant on the great circle $E(\omega_*)$, and Lemma 2.1.5 is proved. □

Since the sets $\varphi^{-1}(\pi a)$ and $\varphi^{-1}(\pi p/q)$ are contained in Σ both for irrational a and for integers p and q, Lemma 2.1.4 is proved as well. □

Corollary 2.1.2. If convex compact bodies $V_1, V_2 \subset \mathbb{R}^3$ satisfy the assumptions of Theorem 2.1.1, the function $\varphi(\omega)$ is not constant and the set $\varphi^{-1}(0)$ (or $\varphi^{-1}(\pi)$) is a great circle on the sphere S^2, then these bodies V_1 and V_2 have constant width.

Now, we finish the proof of Theorem 2.1.1. Denote by P the plane that contains this great circle. Let P_1 and P_2 be the support planes to the body V_2 parallel to the plane P. Since this convex body has constant width, the common points $x_1 = V_2 \cap P_1$ and $x_2 = V_2 \cap P_2$ belong to the common perpendicular to these planes. Hence, the compact body V_1 has a parallel translate V_1' tangent to the planes P_1 and P_2 at the points x_1 and x_2, respectively. The projections of the bodies V_1' and V_2 in the directions of the vectors from the set $\varphi^{-1}(0)$ coincide and this preimage $\varphi^{-1}(0)$ intersects all the great circles on the sphere S^2. Therefore, for the plane set $\varphi^{-1}(0)$ (or $\varphi^{-1}(\pi)$) Theorem 2.1.1 follows from Süss's lemma and from Lemma 2.1.4. □

Theorem 2.1.2. *If V_1 and V_2 are compact convex bodies in $\mathbb{R}^n$, $n > 2$, such that for any two-dimensional plane $P^2 \subset \mathbb{R}^n$ their projections $V_1(P^2)$ and $V_2(P^2)$ are $SO(2)$-congruent and have no $SO(2)$-symmetries, then V_1 and V_2 are either parallel or centrally symmetric to each other in $\mathbb{R}^n$.*

Proof. For $n > 3$, this theorem is proved by induction on the dimension n. In any Euclidean space $\mathbb{R}^n$ projection of a body V onto any two-dimensional plane P^2 can be done in two steps: first, we project V onto some three-dimensional plane P^3 that contains P^2, and then we project this projection onto P^2. It follows from the previous arguments that the projections of V_1 and V_2 onto any three-dimensional plane in $\mathbb{R}^n$ are either parallel or centrally symmetric to each other. The type of this transformation is the same for all three-dimensional planes, since the projections of these bodies onto any two-dimensional plane have no $SO(2)$-symmetry. The induction step is based on Süss's lemma. □

Let us note that in all results of this section the projection data cannot be made substantially smaller. Namely, fix some small $\varepsilon > 0$ and denote by D the set of all unit vectors in $S^2 \subset \mathbb{R}^3$ that make angles larger than ε with the vectors $\pm e_3 = (0; 0; \pm 1)$.

Consider the point $N(-0.6; 0.8; 0)$ on the equatorial great circle $E(e_3)$ and two sequences of points $M_i^0(\cos\varphi_i; \sin\varphi_i; 0)$ and $M_i^1(-\cos\varphi_i; -\sin\varphi_i; 0)$, where for all $i \geq 0$ $\varphi_i \in (\pi/6, \pi/4)$, $\varphi_i > \varphi_{i+1}$.

Let $S(M_i^0)$ and $S(M_i^1)$ be symmetric spherical segments of small volumes that are obtained by intersecting the unit ball B with the planes orthogonal to the vectors OM_i^0 and OM_i^1, respectively, and that have their vertices at the points M_i^0, M_i^1. Let $S(N)$ denote a spherical segment of small volume cut from B by the plane orthogonal to the vector ON. The sizes of all segments described above should be small enough to ensure that for any $\omega \in D$ each circle of the great circle $E(\omega)$ intersects the surface of at most one of the segments $S(M_i^0)$, $S(M_i^1)$ or $S(N)$. It is clear that if such a circle intersects $S(M_n^1)$, then it also intersects the symmetric segment $S(M_n^0)$, and also that the segments $S(M_n^1)$ are disjoint and their volumes tend to zero as i increases. All the above means that any plane which contains the origin and makes an angle larger than ε with the horizontal plane intersects either the segment $S(N)$ or a pair of segments $S(M_i^0)$, $S(M_i^1)$ for some $i \geq 0$ or does not intersect any of these segments.

Let Δ be an arbitrary countable sequence of zeros and ones, indexed by natural numbers; it is known that the set of all such sequences has power of continuum. Let V_Δ denote the convex compact set obtained from the ball B by removing the segments $S(N)$, $S(M_0^1)$ and the segments $S(M_i^\alpha)$, $i \geq 1$, where α equals 0 or 1, according to the following rule: if the ith position in the sequence Δ is occupied by 0 or 1, respectively, then we remove $S(M_i^0)$ or $S(M_i^1)$, respectively.

Clearly, the convex compact sets V_Δ are pairwise noncongruent, but their projections along any vector in D are congruent. In fact, if we suppose that for such a vector ω the circle $E(\omega)$ intersects the surface of the segments $S(N)$ and $S(M_0^1)$ or does not intersect any of the segments constructed above, then the projections of all V_Δ along ω coincide. If the circle $E(\omega)$ intersects a pair of segments $S(M_i^1)$ and $S(M_i^0)$, $i \geq 1$, then the projections of all V_Δ along ω either coincide or are centrally symmetric to each other, depending on whether there is 0 or 1 in the ith position of the sequence Δ. Naturally, the projections of the sets V_Δ along vectors that are sufficiently close to $\pm e_3$ are not necessarily congruent, but the measure of the set of such directions, which depends on ε, can be made as small as desired. It is not difficult to see that for any $\omega \in S^2$ the areas $S(V_\Delta(\omega))$ and the perimeters $L(V_\Delta(\omega))$ of the projections of the convex compact sets V_Δ depend only on the projection ω and not on Δ.

A similar purely algebraic example will be constructed in Section 3.3.

For two convex compact bodies as above, consider the lengths of their chords containing some fixed points. Using the methods developed in this section and the polar duality construction, one can obtain an analogue of Theorem 2.1.1:

Theorem 2.1.3. *Let $V_1, V_2 \subset \mathbb{R}^n$, $n > 2$, be convex compact bodies and $q_i \in V_i$ be their interior points. If the sections of these bodies given by parallel two-dimensional planes containing q_1 and q_2 are $SO(2)$-congruent and have no $SO(2)$-symmetries, and these points q_1 and q_2 correspond to each other in such congruences, then the bodies V_1 and V_2 are either parallel-translation equivalent or centrally symmetric to each other in $\mathbb{R}^n$.*

Proof. The proof follows that of Theorem 2.1.1 almost literally: we start with the case $n = 3$ and suppose from the very beginning that $q_1 = q_2 = q$ after some parallel translation of V_1. Denote by $P(\omega)$ an oriented plane containing q and orthogonal to $\omega \in S^2$ and by $V_i(\omega)$ the corresponding sections of V_i as above. The angle $\varphi(\omega)$ of rotation of $V_1(\omega)$ to $V_2(\omega)$ depends on ω continuously because of the asymmetry of the sections. As in the proof of Theorem 2.1.1, one of the preimages $\varphi^{-1}(0)$, $\varphi^{-1}(\pi) \subset S^2$ intersects all the meridians of this unit sphere. If it is $\varphi^{-1}(0)$, then one can verify that $V_1 = V_2$; if it is $\varphi^{-1}(\pi)$, then V_1 is centrally symmetric to V_2 and q is the center of this symmetry. The case $n > 3$ follows from Süss's lemma. □

2.2. AN ATTEMPT TO RELAX THE ASYMMETRY CONDITIONS

In the previous section we have obtained a collection of results on the uniqueness of recovering the shapes of convex bodies from the shapes of their projections onto two-dimensional planes. The condition of the absence of $SO(2)$-symmetries of these projections, which we have required there, is connected with our topological approach and does not seem to be quite natural from the geometrical viewpoint of our Main Question: If two bodies have congruent projection onto any plane, how different can they be? The author still has no definite idea whether this asymmetry condition is essential in Theorems 2.1.1 and 2.1.2.

Here we shall describe one attempt to omit this condition, and the main result that we have managed to obtain in this direction is

Theorem 2.2.1. *If compact convex bodies V_1 and V_2 in $\mathbb{R}^n$, $n > 2$, have twice continuously differentiable support functions and for any two-dimensional plane $P^2 \subset \mathbb{R}^n$ their projections $V_1(P^2)$ and $V_2(P^2)$ are $SO(2)$-congruent and*

either are disks,

or have no constant width,

or have no $SO(2)$-symmetries,

then the bodies V_1 and V_2 are either parallel or centrally symmetric to each other.

Proof. As in the previous sections, we begin with the consideration of the case $n = 3$. The higher-dimensional variants of this theorem easily follow by induction as in our previous theorems.

It is clear that a figure of constant width having $SO(2)$-symmetry of even order is centrally symmetric and hence is a disk. Under the assumptions of the theorem, all the noncircular projections of constant width have no $SO(2)$-symmetries. It follows from the proof of Lemma 2.1.1 that on each connected component of the open set $\Psi = S^2 \backslash (\varphi^{-1}(0) \cup \varphi^{-1}(\pi))$ the function $\varphi(\omega)$ is continuous. We remind that according to Lemma 2.1.1, $\Psi \subset \Sigma$, i. e., for any $\omega \in \Psi$ the projections $V_1(\omega)$ and $V_2(\omega)$ have constant width.

For the proof of the theorem, we consider three cases:

a. In the very special case when Ψ is empty and $S^2 \backslash \varphi^{-1}(0)$ is nonempty, if all meridians of the unit sphere that have endpoints $\pm\omega_1 \in S^2 \setminus \varphi^{-1}(0)$ intersect the preimage $\varphi^{-1}(0)$ (where $0 \neq \varphi(\omega_1) \neq \pi$, as in the previous section), then

(i) if $\varphi^{-1}(0)$ is a great circle, we have $\varphi^{-1}(\pi) = S^2$ and Süss's lemma implies that in this case V_1 and V_2 are centrally symmetric to each other;

(ii) if $\varphi^{-1}(0)$ is not a great circle, then it follows from the results of Section 2.1 that $\varphi(\omega_1) = 0$, which contradicts the choice of ω_1. If one of these meridians, say m (and all meridians close to it), does not intersect the closed set $\varphi^{-1}(0)$, then some neighborhood M of the great circle containing the meridian m is contained in $\varphi^{-1}(\pi)$. As in Section 2.1, we change the body V_1 for the body V_1'' centrally symmetric to V_1 with respect to an appropriate point so that, as above, for all $\omega \in S^2$ the projections $V_1''(\omega)$ and $V_2(\omega)$ coincide. Therefore, $V_2 = V_1''$ and consequently $V_2 = V_1$ are centrally symmetric to each other.

b. Now, let ω_2 be a point of the nonempty set Ψ such that $\varphi(\omega_2) = \pi \cdot a$, where a is irrational.

By the assumptions of the theorem, the function $\varphi(\omega)$ is uniquely determined and therefore it is continuous in the domain $\Sigma \setminus (\varphi^{-1}(0) \cup \varphi^{-1}(\pi))$; hence, this function is odd in this domain. It follows from Lemma 2.1.2 that any curve on the unit sphere with endpoints $\pm\omega_2$ intersects $\varphi^{-1}(0) \cup \varphi^{-1}(\pi)$ and also $[\varphi^{-1}(0)] \cup [\varphi^{-1}(\pi)]$. Hence, the great circle $E(\omega_2)$ orthogonal to ω_2 can be represented as a union $E(\omega_2) = A_0 \cup A_\pi$, where A_0 consists of those unit vectors ψ for which there exists a vector $\omega(\psi) \in [\varphi^{-1}(0)]$ orthogonal to ψ and any $\psi \in A_\pi$ is orthogonal to some vector from $[\varphi^{-1}(\pi)]$.

If all meridians $m(\omega_2, \psi)$ with endpoints $\pm\omega_2$ on S^2 parametrized by the "longitude" $\psi \in [0, 2\pi)$ intersect the preimage $\varphi^{-1}(0)$ (or $\varphi^{-1}(\pi)$), then, as in Section 2.1, it can be shown that the bodies V_1 and V_2 are parallel (or, respectively, centrally symmetric to each other). Now we consider the case when some of these meridians do not intersect the preimage $\varphi^{-1}(0)$ and some of them do not intersect $\varphi^{-1}(\pi)$.

Lemma 2.2.1. *If $\varphi^{-1}(0)$ does not lie in a great circle, then the body V_1 is parallel to some V_1' such that the projections of V_2 and V_1' along all vectors in $\varphi^{-1}(0)$ coincide.*

Proof. Let us choose three noncoplanar vectors in $\varphi^{-1}(0)$, as in Lemma 1.2.2. Then our lemma becomes obvious. □

Lemma 2.2.2. *If $\varphi^{-1}(\pi)$ does not intersect all meridians $m(\omega_2, \psi)$, then the body V_1 is parallel to some V_1' such that the projections of V_2 and V_1' along all vectors in $\varphi^{-1}(0)$ coincide.*

Proof. In view of the previous lemma, it is sufficient to examine the case when $\varphi^{-1}(0)$ lies on some great circle. By the assumptions, the preimage $\varphi^{-1}(0)$ is not contained in $\varphi^{-1}(\pi)$. From Lemma 2.1.4 it follows that for all $\omega \in \varphi^{-1}(0) \setminus (\varphi^{-1}(0) \cap \varphi^{-1}(\pi))$ the projections $V_1(\omega)$ and $V_2(\omega)$ have constant width. Let us denote by ω_0 the unit vector orthogonal to the plane containing $\varphi^{-1}(0)$, and let us consider the body V_1' parallel to V_1 such that the points of the boundaries $\partial V_1'$ and ∂V_2 with outward normals $\pm\omega_0$ coincide. By the definition of ω_0, this body V_1' does exist. It is clear that for such a pair of convex bodies V_1' and V_2 their projections along all vectors in $\varphi^{-1}(0)$ coincide, which is required. □

If we consider the body V_1'' centrally symmetric to V_1 instead of V_1, then the closed centrally symmetric sets A_0 and A_π change their roles in the same way as $\varphi^{-1}(0)$ and $\varphi^{-1}(\pi)$, i. e., $A_0'' = A_\pi$ and $A_\pi'' = A_0$.

If the set A_π is dense in the great circle $E(\omega_2)$, then it follows from Theorem 2.1.1 that the bodies V_1 and V_2 are centrally symmetric to each other. Thus, we can assume that the set A_0 contains an open arc L_0 which is not contained in A_π, and A_π contains an open arc L_π which is not contained in A_0. Let V_1' be as in the previous two lemmas.

Lemma 2.2.3. *The points of the boundaries $\partial V_1'(\omega_2)$ and $\partial V_2(\omega_2)$ with the outward normals in A_0 coincide.*

Proof. Let $M_1 \neq M_2$ be disjoint points of these boundaries $M_1 \in \partial V_1'(\omega_2)$ and $M_2 \in \partial V_2(\omega_2)$ such that the corresponding normal vectors $\nu(M_1)$ and $\nu(M_2)$ to $\partial V_1'(\omega_2)$ and $\partial V_2(\omega_2)$ coincide. Let $N_1 \in \partial V_1'$ and $N_2 \in \partial V_2$ be the preimages of M_1 and M_2, respectively, under the projection along ω_2. Since for all ω close to ω_2 the projections $\partial V_1'(\omega)$ and $\partial V_2(\omega)$ are figures of constant width and therefore are strictly convex, each of the points M_1 and M_2 has a unique preimage, N_1 and N_2, respectively. It is clear that the point N_1 with some neighborhood $U_1 \subset \partial V_1'$ does not lie in V_2, while N_2 together with some neighborhood $U_2 \subset \partial V_2$ does not lie in V_1'.

In the plane orthogonal to $\nu(M_1) = \nu(M_2)$ there is a vector $\alpha_0 \in [\varphi^{-1}(0)]$ such that the projections of the points N_1 and N_2 along α_0 coincide on $\partial V_1'(\alpha_0) = \partial V_2(\alpha_0)$. For definiteness assume that the vector $\overrightarrow{N_1N_2}$ has the same direction as α_0. The images of the neighborhoods U_1 and U_2 under the projections along the vectors close to α_0 in $[\varphi^{-1}(0)]$ will not intersect each other, just like under the projection along the vector α_0. If $\alpha \in [\varphi^{-1}(0)]$ is sufficiently close to α_0 but not equal to it, and orthogonal to $\nu(M_1)$, then the projections $V_1'(\alpha)$ and $V_1(\alpha)$ do not coincide, since the projection of N_1 will not lie in $V_2(\alpha)$ and the projection of N_2 will not lie in $V_1'(\alpha)$. If the angle between α and $\nu(M_1)$ is obtuse, then the projection of the neighborhood U_1 along α does not intersect $V_2(\alpha)$, and if this angle is acute, then the projection of the neighborhood U_2 along α does not intersect $V_1'(\alpha)$. Hence, the assumptions of the existence of a pair of points $M_1 \neq M_2$ leads us to a contradiction. □

Lemma 2.2.4. *The set of points in $\partial V_1'(\omega_2) \cap \partial V_2(\omega_2)$ with outward normals in $A_0 \cap A_\pi$ is centrally symmetric.*

Proof. We perform a parallel translation of the body V_1'' considered above so that for the obtained body V_1''' the boundary points of the projection $\partial V_1'''(\omega_2)$ with outward normals in $A_\pi = A_0'''$ coincide with the corresponding points of the projection $\partial V_2(\omega_2)$. The projections $V_1'''(\omega_2)$ and $V_1'(\omega_2)$ are centrally symmetric to each other with respect to reflection at some point O; thus the set of the points in $\partial V_1'(\omega_2) \cap \partial V_2(\omega_2)$ with outward normals in the intersection $A_0 \cap A_\pi$ is centrally symmetric with respect to the same point O, which is required. □

Now, let w be the width of the figures $V_1(\omega_2)$ and $V_1'(\omega_2)$. For any $\psi \in A_0$, the support functions of these figures of constant width coincide. If $\psi_1 \in A_\pi = A_0'''$ and the support functions $H(V_1(\omega_2))(\psi_1) = H(V_2(\omega_2))(-\psi_1)$ are defined with respect to the point O from the previous lemma, then

$$H(V_1'(\omega_2))(\psi_1) = H(V_2(\omega_2))(-\psi_1)$$

and thus

$$H(V_1'(\omega_2))(\psi_1) + H(V_2(\omega_2))(-\psi_1) = w.$$

The points of the boundary $\partial V_1'(\omega_2)$ whose outward normals belong to the arc L_0 lie on the boundary $\partial V_2(\omega_2)$ as well. Therefore, for all $\psi_0 \in L_0$ the points of the boundaries $\partial V_1'(\omega_2)$ and $\partial V_2(\omega_2)$ with outward normals ψ_0 coincide and have the same curvatures. We remind that under the hypothesis of the theorem the support functions of the bodies V_1 and V_2 are twice continuously differentiable. If χ belongs to $(E(\omega_2) \setminus A_0) \subset A_\pi$, then, by the definition of the set A_π, we have $R_1(-\chi) = R_2(\chi)$, where $R_i(\alpha)$ is the curvature radius of the boundary $\partial V_i(\omega_2)$ of the projection at the point with outward normal α; here $i = 1, 2$. Since for the figures of constant width w one has $R_i(\alpha) + R_i(-\alpha) = w$ (see, for example, Egglestone 1958), we obtain $R_1(\chi) + R_2(\chi) = w$ for $\chi \in (E(\omega_2) \setminus A_0)$.

Let R_0 be the curvature radius of $\partial V_1'(\omega_2)$ at the point with outward normal ψ_0. Then $R_1(-\psi_0) = w - R_0$. On this boundary, we consider the pairs of antipodal points with outward normals $\pm\psi_k$ obtained from the vectors $\pm\psi_0$ by rotations through the angles $k\pi \cdot a$. If $\psi_k \in (E(\omega_2)\backslash A_\pi)$, then the radii of curvature of $\partial V_1'(\omega_2)$ and $\partial V_2(\omega_2)$ at the points with outward normals $\pm\psi_k$ coincide. If $\psi_k \in (E(\omega_2) \setminus \mathrm{A}_0)$, then the sum of the curvature radii equals w at such points.

If $A_0 \cap A_\pi$ is nowhere dense, then by rotating it through the angles $k\pi \cdot a$ we obtain nowhere dense sets $(A_0 \cap A_\pi)_k$. The countable union of these intersections, according to Baire's theorem, has dense complement $D \subset E(\omega_2)$, and the sequence of the unit vectors $\pm\psi_k$ can be constructed in this complement D.

If $A_0 \cap A_\pi$ is dense in an open centrally symmetric interval $I \subset E(\omega_2)$, then the curvature radii of the boundaries $\partial V_1(\omega_2)$ and $\partial V_2(\omega_2)$ of the projections at the points with outward normals from this interval I are equal to $w/2$. Let $I_k \subset E(\omega_2)$, $k = 1, 2 \ldots$, be obtained from I by rotation through the angles $k\pi \cdot a$. Suppose that for the points of $\partial V_2(\omega_2)$ with outward normals from the intervals I_s, where $s \leq m-1$, the curvature radii are equal to $w/2$ and to the corresponding curvature radii of the boundary $\partial V_1'(\omega_2)$. Then we perform the inductive step: for the points of $\partial V_2(\omega_2)$ with outward normals in I_m the curvature radii are also equal to $w/2$ because these points are obtained from the corresponding points of $\partial V_1'(\omega_2)$ with outward normals in the interval I_{m-1} by rotation through the angle $\pi \cdot a$. From the relation $R_1(\chi) = R_2(\pm\chi)$ and the continuity of the functions $R_1(\psi)$ and $R_2(\psi)$, it follows that the curvature radii at the points of $\partial V_1'(\omega_2)$ with outward normals from I_m are also equal to $w/2$, since the sets A_0 and A_π are closed. The union of all intervals I_k covers the entire great circle $E(\omega_2)$; hence, both of the projections $\partial V_1'(\omega_2)$ and $\partial V_2(\omega_2)$ are circles with radius $w/2$.

And finally, when the vectors $\pm\psi_k$ do not belong to the countable union of $(A_0 \cap A_\pi)_k$ but densely cover the great circle $E(\omega_2)$, it follows from the continuity of the functions $R_i(\psi)$, $i = 1, 2$, that $R_0 = w - R_0$ and that the boundaries $\partial V_i(\omega_2)$ are circles. Hence, $\omega_2 \in \varphi^{-1}(0) \cap \varphi^{-1}(\pi) \cap \Sigma$, which contradicts the irrationality of $\varphi(\omega_2)/\pi$.

The assumption of the smoothness of the support functions of the bodies V_1 and V_2 was used only in the arguments concerning the curvature of the boundaries of the projections.

c. Now, let us consider the last case when all the quotients $\varphi(\omega)/\pi$ are rational. For each connected component $\Psi^{(j)}$ of the set $\Psi \subset S^2$, let the function $\varphi(\omega)$ be constant and equal to $\pi \cdot r^{(j)}$, where $r^{(j)}$ is rational. Let

$\varphi(\Psi^{(1)}) = \pi p/q$, and $\partial\Psi^{(1)} \subset \varphi^{-1}(0) \cup \varphi^{-1}(\pi)$. Suppose that $0 \neq p \neq q$, since the case $S^2 = \varphi^{-1}(0) \cup \varphi^{-1}(\pi)$ was considered above. For any boundary point $\omega_3 \in \partial\Psi^{(1)}$, the projections $V_i(\omega_3)$ are congruent with respect to

1. rotation through the angle $\pi p/q$ and, at the same time,

2. rotation through the angle 0 or π depending on whether ω_3 belongs to $\varphi^{-1}(0)$ or $\varphi^{-1}(\pi)$.

Since $\omega_3 \subset \Sigma$ and the projections $V_i(\omega_3)$ are congruent with respect to rotations through different angles, i.e., they have no $SO(2)$-symmetries, under the assumptions of our theorem these projections can be only disks that are parallel-translation equivalent. Hence, on the boundary $\partial\Psi^{(1)}$ zero is one of the values of the multivalued function $\varphi(\omega)$ and on each meridian connecting the points $\pm\omega_2 \in \Psi$ there are points from the set $\varphi^{-1}(0)$, and on almost all such meridians there are points from the set $[\varphi^{-1}(0)]$, which implies the coincidence of the great circle $E(\omega_2)$ and the set A_0. It follows from Lemma 2.2.3 that $V_1'(\omega_2) = V_2(\omega_2)$, which contradicts the choice of the vector $\omega_2 \in S^2 \setminus (\varphi^{-1}(0) \cup \varphi^{-1}(\pi))$. □

Theorem 2.2.1 is proved, but this is not the expected perfect result because now we require that the noncircular projections of constant width should not have $SO(2)$-symmetries. Clearly, it is difficult to fix a convex piece of wet soap in the hand, especially if it has constant width.

On the other hand, if convex bodies $V_1, V_2 \subset \mathbb{R}^3$ are polyhedrons and their projections onto any plane are $SO(2)$-congruent, then for any unit $\omega \in S^2$ the projections $V_1(\omega)$ and $V_2(\omega)$ have equal numbers of vertices. From this coincidence only, it is not difficult to deduce that for any face $F_1^{(j)}$ of V_1 there exists a face $F_2^{(j)}$ of V_2 and that this correspondence is one-to-one. Similar isomorphism exists for the edges of these polyhedrons. A. D. Aleksandov (1937) called such polyhedrons analogous. Now, taking into account the $SO(2)$-congruence of their projections, one can verify that V_1 and V_2 are either parallel or centrally symmetric to each other without any additional assumptions on the asymmetry of their projections. A similar statement holds in the case of higher dimension.

2.3. THE CASE OF $(n-2)$-VISIBLE AND $(n-2)$-CONVEX BODIES

This section is devoted to some generalizations of the results of Sections 1.2 and 2.1, in particular, Theorems 2.1.1 and 2.1.2, to wider classes of multidimensional objects in Euclidean spaces, i. e., to the classes of $(n-2)$-visible and $(n-2)$-convex bodies.

Theorem 2.3.1. *Let $W_1, W_2 \subset \mathbb{R}^n$, $n \geq 3$, be compact $(n-2)$-convex bodies such that*

(1) for any two-dimensional plane $P^2 \subset \mathbb{R}^n$, their projections $W_1(P^2)$ and $W_2(P^2)$ are $SO(2)$-congruent and

(2) the convex hulls of these projections have no $SO(2)$-symmetries.

Then W_1 and W_2 are either parallel or centrally symmetric to each other in $\mathbb{R}^n$.

Proof. Since the convex hulls $\operatorname{conv} W_1$ and $\operatorname{conv} W_2$ of the bodies W_1 and W_2 have $SO(2)$-congruent projections onto any two-dimensional plane, it follows from Theorem 2.1.2 that these convex hulls are congruent with respect to either a parallel translation T or a central symmetry S. Suppose that this transformation $F = T$ or S is not a congruence of the bodies W_1 and W_2, say, $F(W_1) \neq W_2$, while $F(\operatorname{conv} W_1) = \operatorname{conv} W_2$, and that some point $M \in F(W_1)$ is not contained in W_2 (or vice versa). Consider any $(n-2)$-dimensional plane P containing this point M and disjoint from W_2. Let Q^2 be the orthogonal complement of P in $\mathbb{R}^n$. The projections of the $(n-2)$-convex bodies $F(W_1)$ and W_2 onto Q^2 are $SO(2)$-congruent and the convex hulls of these projections coincide. Therefore, the projection of $F(W_1)$ onto Q^2 can be obtained from the corresponding projection of W_2 neither by a nonzero translation nor by a rotation, since the convex hulls of these projections have no $SO(2)$-symmetries. This contradicts the existence of the point M. $\square$

Theorem 2.3.2. *Let $W_1, W_2 \subset \mathbb{R}^n$, $n \geq 3$, be compact $(n-2)$-visible simply connected bodies such that*

(1) for any two-dimensional plane $P^2 \subset \mathbb{R}^n$, their projections $W_1(P^2)$ and $W_2(P^2)$ are $SO(2)$-congruent and

(2) have no $SO(2)$-symmetries.

Then W_1 and W_2 are either parallel or centrally symmetric to each other in $\mathbb{R}^n$.

Proof. First, we consider the case $n = 3$. As in the previous section, since for all $\omega \in S^2$ the projections $W_1(\omega)$ and $W_2(\omega)$ have no $SO(2)$-symmetries, we can define a continuous function $\varphi(\omega)$.

It follows from the uniqueness of solutions of the integral equation (2.1.1) that the width functions of the convex hulls $\operatorname{conv} W_1$ and $\operatorname{conv} W_2$ coincide in all directions.

If $0 \neq \varphi(\omega_0) \neq \pi$ for some $\omega_0 \in S^2$ and $\varphi(\omega) \neq \text{const}$ in any neighborhood of ω_0 on the sphere, then in any such neighborhood of this vector there are unit vectors ω for which the quotients $\varphi(\omega)/\pi$ are irrational. Hence, the convex hulls of the projections $\operatorname{conv} W_1(\omega_0)$ and $\operatorname{conv} W_2(\omega_0)$ have constant widths.

Lemma 2.3.1. *For any point in the boundaries of the projections* $\operatorname{conv} W_1(\omega_0)$ *or* $\operatorname{conv} W_2(\omega_0)$*, its preimage with respect to the projection in the direction* ω_0 *on the boundary* $\partial \operatorname{conv} W_1$ *or* $\partial \operatorname{conv} W_2$*, respectively, consists of a single point.*

Proof. For all ω sufficiently close to ω_0, the corresponding projections $\operatorname{conv} W_1(\omega)$ and $\operatorname{conv} W_2(\omega)$ have the same constant width as well.

If the indicated preimage contains an interval, then this interval should be seen on the boundaries of some projections $\operatorname{conv} W_1(\omega_1)$ and $\operatorname{conv} W_2(\omega_1)$ for some ω_1 close to ω_0, but these projections should have constant width, as it was noted above. □

It follows from the uniqueness of these preimages that the preimages of the strictly convex boundaries $\operatorname{conv} W_1(\omega_0)$ and $\operatorname{conv} W_2(\omega_0)$ are closed lines on the boundaries of the compact bodies W_1 and W_2. Since these bodies are simply connected, the boundaries $\operatorname{conv} W_1(\omega_0)$ and $\operatorname{conv} W_2(\omega_0)$ are homotopic to zero in the projections $W_1(\omega_0)$ and $W_2(\omega_0)$, respectively. Hence, these projections $W_1(\omega_0)$ and $W_2(\omega_0)$ are convex, have constant width and have no $SO(2)$-symmetries: $\operatorname{conv} W_i(\omega_0) = W_i(\omega_0)$, $i = 1, 2$. It follows from Lemma 1.2.6 that the convex hulls $\operatorname{conv} W_1$ and $\operatorname{conv} W_2$ are either parallel or centrally symmetric to each other; therefore, the projection $W_1(\omega_0) = \operatorname{conv} W_1(\omega_0)$ is obtained from $W_2(\omega_0)$ by the same transformation, which contradicts the choice of ω_0.

Now, we shall consider the higher-dimensional cases of Theorem 2.3.2. In contrast with the previous Theorem 2.3.1, the projections of convex hulls of the bodies W_1 and W_2 onto two-dimensional planes can have $SO(2)$-symmetries. The inductive step of the proof is based on the fact that the projection of a q-visible compact body in $\mathbb{R}^n$ onto any hyperplane is $(q-1)$-visible.

Indeed, assume that for the Euclidean space $\mathbb{R}^{n-1}$ this theorem is established. Note that the projection of any object in $\mathbb{R}^n$ onto a two-dimensional plane $P^2 \subset P^{n-1}$ can be realized in two steps:

first, onto the hyperplane P^{n-1},

and then from P^{n-1} onto P^2.

The projections of the bodies W_1 and W_2 onto any hyperplane are either parallel or centrally symmetric to each other. Moreover, if the projections of W_1 and W_2 onto a hyperplane P_1^{n-1} are parallel and projections onto another hyperplane P_2^{n-1} are centrally symmetric to each other, then their projections onto the intersection $P_1^{n-1} \cap P_2^{n-1}$ should have $SO(2)$-symmetry, because they are congruent with respect to two different transformations. So, we complete the inductive step with the help of Süss's lemma. □

It is worth emphasizing that these two theorems are not consequences of each other, since the conditions (1) and (2) of Theorem 2.3.2 are stronger than the corresponding conditions of Theorem 2.3.1; on the other hand, not every $(n-2)$-convex body in $\mathbb{R}^n$ is $(n-2)$-visible.

Note that, in contrast with the case of convex bodies, the absence of the $SO(2)$-symmetries is essential for the $(n-2)$-visible and $(n-2)$-convex bodies:

Let $Q = I^3 \cup \Lambda$ be the union of the cube $I^3 \subset \mathbb{R}^3$ and the cone Λ with summit at the point $(-0.5; 0.5; 1.1)$ and base $z = 1$, $(x+0.5)^2 + (y-0.5)^2 = 0.01$. We set

$$G_1 = \{(x,y,z) \mid [0.6 < x < 0.7; y > 0.8] \text{ or } [-0.7 < x < -0.6; z > 1.8 + y] \\ \text{or } [-0.7 < x < -0.6; z > -1.8 - y]\}$$

and

$$G_2 = \{(x,y,z) \mid [0.6 < x < 0.7; z > 1.8 - y] \text{ or } [0.6 < x < 0.7; z > y - 1.8] \\ \text{or } [-0.7 < x < -0.6; y < -0.8]\}.$$

Let $W_1 = Q \setminus G_1$ and $W_2 = Q \setminus G_2$ (see Figure 2.2).

Clearly, these bodies W_1 and W_2 are 1-visible in $\mathbb{R}^3$ and are not congruent or even affinely equivalent to each other. On the other hand, their projections onto "almost vertical" planes, i. e., where the cone Λ is seen on the projection and the sets $J_\pm = [0.6 < |x| < 0.7; |y| > 0.8]$ are not seen through, coincide. In this case $\varphi(\omega) = 0$.

Their projections onto "almost horizontal" planes, where the cone Λ is not seen while the sets $J_\pm$ are seen through, are pairwise centrally symmetric to each other; here $\varphi(\omega) = \pi$. Between these two cases there are sufficiently many directions $\omega = (\omega_x, \omega_y, \omega_z)$ such that $0.2 < |\omega_z| < 0.5$.

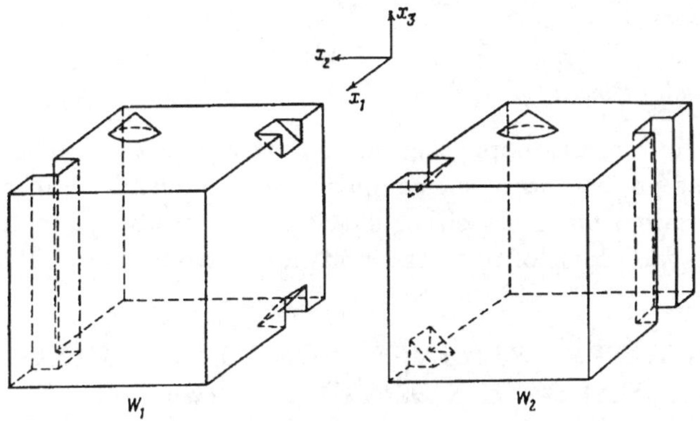

Figure 2.2: Visible bodies W_1 and W_2

The corresponding projections $W_1(\omega)$ and $W_2(\omega)$ coincide and have central symmetry, thus, the rotation angle $\varphi(\omega)$ cannot be well defined. An analogous counterexample with nontrivial fundamental group was constructed by A. V. Kuz'minykh.

Theorems 2.3.1 and 2.3.2 can be formulated in the infinite-dimensional case as well.

Definition. A compact body W in a separable Hilbert space $\mathcal{H}$ will be called $(-q)$-*visible* if any plane of codimension greater than q that is disjoint from W is contained in some plane of codimension q that is disjoint from W as well.

Definition. A compact body W in a separable Hilbert space $\mathcal{H}$ will be called $(-q)$-*convex* if for every point $x \notin W$ there is a plane of codimension q that contains x and is disjoint from W.

Theorem 2.3.3. *Let $W_1, W_2 \subset \mathcal{H}$ be compact (-2)-convex bodies. If their projections $W_1(P^2)$ and $W_2(P^2)$ onto any two-dimensional plane $P^2 \subset \mathcal{H}$ are $SO(2)$-congruent and the convex hulls of these projections have no $SO(2)$-symmetries, then W_1 and W_2 are either parallel or centrally symmetric to each other in $\mathcal{H}$.*

Theorem 2.3.4. *Let $W_1, W_2 \subset \mathcal{H}$ be compact (-2)-visible simply connected bodies. If their projections $W_1(P^2)$ and $W_2(P^2)$ onto* *any two-dimensional plane $P^2 \subset \mathcal{H}$ are $SO(2)$-congruent and have no $SO(2)$-symmetries, then W_1 and W_2 are either parallel or centrally symmetric to each other in $\mathcal{H}$.*

Our previous results imply that under the assumptions of Theorems 2.3.3 and 2.3.4 the projections of the compact bodies W_1 and W_2 in $\mathcal{H}$ onto any finite-dimensional plane are either parallel or centrally symmetric to each other. Then the proofs of these theorems follow from Lemma 1.2.8.

2.4. STABILITY ESTIMATES FOR RECOVERING THE SHAPES OF CONVEX BODIES FROM THE SHAPES OF THEIR PROJECTIONS

In this section we obtain some stability estimates for the solutions of the reconstruction problems considered above.

Since the main results of this chapter were obtained for the objects whose projections onto all two-dimensional planes do not have $SO(2)$-symmetries, here we shall impose a similar restriction.

A compact convex body $V \subset \mathbb{R}^n$ will be called *admissible* if

(1) *all its projections onto two-dimensional planes have no $SO(2)$-symmetries;*

(2) *all these projections do not have constant width.*

In the sequel we shall denote by $W^{d\varepsilon}$ the $d\varepsilon$-neighborhood of a compact set W whose diameter equals d.

Let $V \subset \mathbb{R}^n$ be a convex compact body. It is obvious that for any $\varepsilon > 0$ there exists an admissible convex body $V' \subset \mathbb{R}^n$ such that $\rho_h(V, V') < d\varepsilon$,

Given a convex admissible body $V_1 \subset \mathbb{R}^n$, let ε_0 be a positive number such that for any two-dimensional plane $P^2 \subset \mathbb{R}^n$ the $d\varepsilon_0$-neighborhood of the boundary $\partial V_1(P^2)$ of the projection of V_1 does not contain closed curves L that have $SO(2)$-symmetry and are $d\varepsilon$-close to $\partial V_1(P^2)$, i. e., $\rho_h(L, \partial V_1(P^2)) < d\varepsilon_0$. The same notation ε_0 will be used later in order to describe sufficiently small neighborhoods of convex figures in $\mathbb{R}^2$ that have no $SO(2)$-symmetries.

Now, we shall study the case of convex bodies in the 3-dimensional Euclidean space. Let SI be the group of the orientation-preserving isometries of a two-dimensional plane. Consider $\varepsilon < \varepsilon_0$ and a convex compact body $V_2 \subset \mathbb{R}^3$ whose projection onto an arbitrary plane $P(\omega)$ is $SO(2)$-congruent to within $d\varepsilon$ to the corresponding projection $V_1(\omega)$, i.e.,

$$\rho_{SI}(V_1(\omega), V_2(\omega)) < d\varepsilon.$$

Denote by $V_2'(\omega) \subset P(\omega)$ the result of such an isometry: $\rho_h(V_1(\omega), V_2'(\omega)) < d\varepsilon$, and let $\{\Phi(\omega)\} \subset S^1$ be the set of all the angles of rotations of $V_2(\omega)$ which transform $V_2(\omega)$ into figures $V_2''(\omega)$ which are parallel to the projection $V_2'(\omega)$. Clearly, choosing an appropriate center of any particular rotation of $V_2(\omega)$ we can obtain $V_2''(\omega) = V_2'(\omega)$, but Süss's lemma and Groemer's estimates (see Definition 1.1.11) allow us to avoid this choice problem.

As in our previous considerations, we shall suppose that all these angles of rotations $\varphi(\omega)$ lie in the segment $[-\pi; \pi]$ with identified endpoints, and in this sense the inequality $|\phi - \pi| < \delta$ implies that either $\pi - \phi < \delta$ or $\phi + \pi < \delta$.

The main aim of the present section is to prove that if all the projections of admissible convex compact bodies $V_1, V_2 \subset \mathbb{R}^3$ are $d\varepsilon$-close for sufficiently small $\varepsilon > 0$ in the sense of the metric ρ_{SI}, then these bodies are either parallel or centrally symmetric to each other to within a Hausdorff distance of order $d\varepsilon^{1/3}$. Namely, the following theorem holds:

Theorem 2.4.1. *Let $V_1 \subset \mathbb{R}^3$ be an admissible compact convex body. Then there exists a positive ε_1 ($\varepsilon_1 \leq \varepsilon_0$) such that if $\varepsilon < \varepsilon_1$ and all the projections of a compact convex body $V_2 \subset \mathbb{R}^3$ onto all planes are $d\varepsilon$-close to the corresponding projections of the body V_1 in the sense of the metric ρ_{SI}, then V_1 and V_2 are either parallel or centrally symmetric to each other to within $3(1+2\sqrt{2})d\varepsilon^{1/3}$ in the sense of the Hausdorff metric.*

Here ε_0 is the number described above just after the definition of admissible convex bodies.

With the help of the estimates established by Groemer (1987) in the case when the projections of V_1 and V_2 are almost parallel, we can obtain the following theorem.

Theorem 2.4.2. *Let $V_1 \subset \mathbb{R}^n$, $n \geq 3$, be an admissible compact convex body. Then there exists a positive ε_1 ($\varepsilon_1 \leq \varepsilon_0$) such that if $\varepsilon < \varepsilon_1$ and all projections of a compact convex body $V_2 \subset \mathbb{R}^n$ onto two-dimensional planes are $d\varepsilon$-close in the sense of the metric ρ_{SI} to the corresponding projections of the body V_1, then the bodies V_1 and V_2 are either parallel or centrally symmetric to each other to within $3(1+2\sqrt{2})^{n-2}d\varepsilon^{1/3}$ in the sense of the Hausdorff metric.*

Proof. This theorem is proved by induction on n. By virtue of the absence of symmetries of the projections of V_1 onto all two-dimensional planes, the projections of V_1 and V_2 onto all hyperplanes, by the previous theorem and the induction hypothesis, are either parallel or centrally symmetric to each other to within the corresponding precision. Therefore, the assertion of the theorem follows from the estimates of Groemer (1987). □

For the proof of Theorem 2.4.1, we need some technical statements whose general meaning is that the sets $\{\Phi(\omega)\}$ of the rotation angles are connected in S^1 for sufficiently small $\varepsilon > 0$.

Lemma 2.4.1. *(Furniture moving). Let $W \subset \mathbb{R}^2$ be a convex compact figure without $SO(2)$-symmetries and let d be its diameter.*

Then there exists $\varepsilon_1 < \varepsilon_0$ such that if $\varepsilon < \varepsilon_1$ and $W' \subset W^{d\varepsilon}$ is $SO(2)$-congruent to W, then W' can be returned continuously to the initial position W inside the $1.5\,d\varepsilon$-neighborhood of W.

Note, that actually we shall see that for sufficiently small ε_1 the coefficient 1.5 can be replaced by an arbitrary coefficient $1+\alpha$, where $\alpha > 0$. The author believes that this continuous movement $W \longleftrightarrow W'$ can be realized inside the $d\varepsilon$-neighborhood of the figure W.

Proof. We fix some $\varepsilon < \varepsilon_0$. In the sequel, if necessary, we shall impose additional restrictions on this ε.

It is obvious that if W' is obtained from W by a parallel translation, then during the inverse translation from W' to W we shall not go out of the neighborhood $W^{d\varepsilon}$. So, we shall assume that the transformation of W to $W' = \varphi(W, O)$ is the rotation through a certain angle φ around a certain center O.

If $O \notin W$ then, with the help of suitable parallel translations of W' inside $W^{d\varepsilon}$, we can reduce our problem to the case when the rotation center O is contained in the interior of W, which we shall consider now. Let us also note that $\varphi \neq \pi$, since otherwise the $d\varepsilon$-neighborhood of the curve ∂W would contain a centrally symmetric curve.

Since ∂W has no $SO(2)$-symmetries, for $\varphi \neq 0$ all the figures $\varphi(W, O)$ do not coincide with the figure W; hence, for $\pi \geq |\varphi| > \varepsilon > 0$ the positive minimum of the translative distances between W and all $\varphi(W, O)$ does exist and satisfies the estimate

$$\min_{\pi \geq |\varphi| > \varepsilon} \rho_t(\varphi(W, O), W) = \varepsilon_2 \cdot d > 0.$$

Here $\varepsilon_2 > 0$ is defined by this equality. Note also that the center O of the rotations does not have any influence on the translative distance ρ_t.

On the other hand, for any center of rotation A we have

$$\varphi \cdot d > \rho_h(\varphi(W, A), W) \geq \rho_t(\varphi(W, A), W).$$

That is why for the angles φ such that $\pi \geq |\varphi| > \varepsilon$ the $\varepsilon_2\, d$-neighborhood of W does not contain any $W' = \varphi(W, O)$, and for $|\varphi| < \varepsilon_2$ any $W' = \varphi(W, O)$ contained in the $\varepsilon_2\, d$-neighborhood of W can be returned to the initial position W inside this neighborhood.

Now, we shall examine the case $\varepsilon_2 < |\varphi| < \varepsilon$, since the case $\varepsilon_2 > \varepsilon$ is very simple because under this assumption any movement from W to W' can be realized inside the corresponding $\varepsilon\, d$-neighborhood of W.

Given $W' = \varphi(W, O) \subset W^{d\varepsilon}$, consider the point $M \in W$ such that the distance $|OM| = R$ is maximal among all the distances $|OX|$, $X \subset W$. As it was noted above, $R < d$. Denote by $M_1 = \varphi(M, O)$ the image of the point M under the rotation by the angle φ around the center O. The chord $\overline{MM_1}$ of the circle which describes this rotation $M \longrightarrow M_1$ is contained in the convex neighborhood $W^{d\varepsilon}$ and the maximal distance from the arc MM_1 of this circle to this chord equals $R \cdot (1 - \cos\varphi/2) = 2R\sin^2\varphi/4 < d \cdot \varphi^2/2$. Hence, the rotation $W' = \varphi(W, O) \longrightarrow W$ can be realized in the $\varepsilon{\cdot}d(1{+}\varepsilon/2)$-neighborhood of the convex figure W. □

Lemma 2.4.2. *Let $W \subset \mathbb{R}^2$ be a convex figure and $\varepsilon_0 > 0$ be as in the preceding lemma. Then, if $\varepsilon < \varepsilon_0$ and for a convex figure W_1 such that $W_1 \subset W^{d\varepsilon}$ there exists $W_1' \subset W^{d\varepsilon}$ which is $SO(2)$-congruent to W_1, then W_1' can be turned into the position W_1 inside the $1.5\, d\varepsilon$-neighborhood of the figure W.*

Proof. Let U be the closure of the $d\varepsilon$-neighborhood of W and U' be the image of U with respect to the SI-isometry of the plane that transforms W_1 into W_1'. Clearly, U' is contained in the $d\varepsilon$-neighborhood of U whose diameter equals $d(1 + 2\varepsilon)$ and, according to the previous lemma, in the $1.4(1 + 2\varepsilon)\, d\varepsilon$-neighborhood of U we can turn U' into the initial position U. The figure W_1' can also be turned into its initial position inside the $1.5\, d\varepsilon$-neighborhood of W_1 together with the neighborhood U'. □

The following lemma can be easily derived from the previous statements.

Lemma 2.4.3. *Under the conditions of Theorem 2.4.1, there exists an $\varepsilon_1 > 0$ ($\varepsilon_1 \leq \varepsilon_0$) such that for all $\varepsilon \leq \varepsilon_1$ and for all $\omega \in S^2$ the set of* *the angles* $\{\Phi(\omega)\} \subset S^1$ *is contained in the segment formed by the angles of rotations which do not bring* $V_2(\omega)$ *outside the boundary of the closure of the* $1.5\, d\varepsilon$*-neighborhood of* $V_1(\omega)$.

We shall denote by $I(\omega, \varepsilon)$ the smallest segment in S^1 that contains $\{\Phi(\omega)\}$.

Proof. Now, we begin the proof of Theorem 2.4.1 step by step.

a.1. If for each unit vector $\omega \in S^2$ the set of angles $\{\Phi(\omega)\}$ contains an angle φ such that $\varphi < \varepsilon^{1/3}$, then for all ω the ρ_t-distance between the projections $V_1(\omega)$ and $V_2(\omega)$ does not exceed $d(\varepsilon + \varepsilon^{1/3})$. It follows from the estimates of Groemer (1987) that in this case the ρ_t-distance between the convex bodies V_1 and $V_2 \subset \mathbb{R}^3$ does not exceed $d(1 + 2\sqrt{2})(\varepsilon + \varepsilon^{1/3})$.

a.2. Analogously, if for each $\omega \in S^2$ the set of angles $\{\Phi(\omega)\}$ contains an angle $\varphi(\omega)$ such that $\pi - |\varphi| < \varepsilon^{1/3}$, we construct a body V_2' that is centrally symmetric to V_2 with respect to a certain point. Then the ρ_t-distance between the bodies V_1 and V_2' does not exceed $d(1 + 2\sqrt{2})(\varepsilon + \varepsilon^{1/3})$. Hence, V_1 and V_2 coincide in $\mathbb{R}^3$ with the same precision after certain central symmetry and after the central symmetries close to it. If $\{\Phi(\omega)\}$ intersects the $\varepsilon^{1/3}$-neighborhood of both angles 0 and π, then the $d(\varepsilon + \varepsilon^{1/3})$-neighborhood of $V_1(\omega)$ contains a centrally symmetric curve, which contradicts the assumptions of the theorem for sufficiently small ε.

Given $\omega_1 \in S^2$, suppose now that the set of angles $\{\Phi(\omega_1)\}$ is contained in the interval $(\varepsilon^{1/3}, \pi - \varepsilon^{1/3})$. We shall denote by N_0 and N_π, respectively, the sets of the unit vectors $\omega_0 \in S^2$ and the unit vectors $\omega_\pi \in S^2$ such that the ρ_t-distance between the projections $V_1(\omega_0)$ and $V_2(\omega_0)$ does not exceed $1.5\, d\varepsilon$ and the projections $V_1(\omega_\pi)$ and $V_2(\omega_\pi)$ are centrally symmetric to each other to within $1.5\, d\varepsilon$. Then, on each meridian joining the endpoints of the vectors $\pm\omega_1$ on the unit sphere, we can find vectors from N_0 or N_π.

This statement follows from the fact that on the unit circle S^1 the sets $\{\Phi(\omega_1)\}$ and $\{\Phi(-\omega_1)\}$, and also the segments $I(\omega_1, \varepsilon)$ and $I(-\omega_1, \varepsilon)$ whose existence has been established in Lemma 2.4.5, are symmetric to each other with respect to the straight line joining the points $0, \pi \in S^1$. During the rotation of the vector ω_1 into the position of $-\omega_1$ along an arbitrary meridian m, the segment $I(\omega, \varepsilon)$ transforms from $I(\omega_1, \varepsilon)$ to $I(-\omega_1, \varepsilon)$, and it is easy to see that $\lim_{\omega \to \omega'} I(\omega, \varepsilon) \subseteq I(\omega', \varepsilon)$. Therefore, $I(\omega, \varepsilon)$ contains the point 0 or the point π of the unit circle for certain $\omega \in m$.

Lemma 2.4.4. *One of the sets* N_0, N_π *intersects all the meridians that join the vectors* $\pm\omega_1 \in S^3$.

Proof. The proof of this lemma repeats that of the corresponding statements of Section 2.1 and is based on the following argument. If a meridian m_1 intersects N_0 and does not intersect N_π, and a meridian m_2 has the opposite property, then there exists a meridian m_3 between them such that any of its neighborhoods contains meridians of types m_1 and m_2. Then there exists a point ω_3 on the meridian m_3 such that the interval $I(\omega_3, \varepsilon)$ intersects both sets N_0 and N_π; hence, the $1.5\,d\varepsilon$-neighborhood of $\partial V_1(\omega_3)$ contains a centrally symmetric curve, which contradicts the assumptions of Theorem 2.4.1 for sufficiently small $\varepsilon > 0$. □

If the set N_π intersects all the meridians, then we consider a central symmetry of the body V_2, and the roles of N_0 and N_π interchange, as in Section 2.1. Therefore, in the sequel we assume that it is the set N_0 that intersects all the meridians above.

b. Denote by $\langle\cdot,\cdot,\cdot\rangle$ the scalar triple product in $\mathbb{R}^3$ and suppose that N_0 contains a triple of vectors β_1, β_2, β_3 such that $|\langle\beta_1,\beta_2,\beta_3\rangle| \geq \varepsilon^{1/3}$. Then it is easily verified that for any vector $\beta \in N_0$ there exist two vectors β_i, β_j in this triple such that $|\langle\beta_1,\beta_2,\beta_3\rangle| \geq \varepsilon^{1/3}/2$.

Let $a(\beta_1) \perp \beta_1$ be a vector such that, after the parallel translation of the body V_2 by this vector, the projection $V_2'(\beta_1)$ of the obtained body V_2' is $1.5\,d\varepsilon$-proximate to the projection $V_1(\beta_1)$ in the sense of the Hausdorff metric. Now consider the vector $a(\beta_2)\perp\beta_2$ of a parallel translation of the body V_2' such that for the obtained body V_2'' the projections $V_2''(\beta_2)$ and $V_1(\beta_2)$ are $1.5\,d\varepsilon$-proximate as above. We claim that the projections $V_2''(\beta_1)$ and $V_1(\beta_1)$ are $3 \cdot 1.5\,d\varepsilon$-proximate. Indeed, denote by $a(\beta_2)(l_{1,2})$ the projection of the vector $a(\beta_2)$ onto the line $l_{1,2} = P(\beta_1) \cap P(\beta_2)$. It is easy to see that the length of this projection does not exceed $3\,d\varepsilon$. Hence, the ρ_h-distance between $V_2''(\beta_2)$ and $V_1(\beta_2)$ does not exceed the sum $\rho_h(V_2''(\beta_2), V_1(\beta_2)) + |a(\beta_2)(l_{1,2})|$.

We superpose the projections $V_1(\beta_1)$ and $V_2(\beta_1)$ to within $1.5\,d\varepsilon$ by a parallel translation of V_2. Then, moving V_2 in the direction of β_1, i. e., without changing its projection along β_1, we can make the projections of $V_1(\beta_2)$ and $V_2(\beta_2)$ proximate to within $4.5\,d\varepsilon$ as well.

Let us estimate the proximity of $V_1(\beta_3)$ and $V_2''(\beta_3)$, obtained by the parallel translation indicated above. Denote by ζ the angle between the straight lines $l_{1,3} = P(\beta_1) \cap P(\beta_3)$ and $l_{2,3} = P(\beta_2) \cap P(\beta_3)$. It is clear that

$$\begin{aligned}|[\beta_1 \times \beta_3]| \cdot |[\beta_2 \times \beta_3]| \cdot \sin\zeta &= |[[\beta_1 \times \beta_3] \times [\beta_2 \times \beta_3]]| \\ &= |\beta_2 \cdot \langle\beta_1,\beta_3,\beta_3\rangle - \beta_3 \cdot \langle\beta_1,\beta_3,\beta_2\rangle| = |\langle\beta_1,\beta_2,\beta_3\rangle| > \varepsilon^{1/3}.\end{aligned}$$

Since the absolute values of the vector products of the unit vectors $|[\beta_i \times \beta_j]|$ do not exceed 1, we have

$$|\sin\zeta| = \frac{|\langle\beta_1, \beta_2, \beta_3\rangle|}{|[\beta_1 \times \beta_3]| \cdot |[\beta_2 \times \beta_3]|} \geq |(\beta_1, \beta_2, \beta_3)| > \varepsilon^{1/3}.$$

As we have shown above, the Hausdorff distances between the projections of V_1 and V_2'' onto the lines $l_{1,3}$ and $l_{2,3}$ do not exceed $4 \cdot 1.5\, d\varepsilon$. Therefore, the length of the vector $a(\beta_3)$ of the parallel translation of V_2'', which makes the Hausdorff distance equal to the translative one, does not exceed

$$\frac{4 \cdot 1.5\, d\varepsilon}{\cos\zeta/2} \leq \frac{6\, d\varepsilon\sqrt{2}}{\sqrt{1 - \sqrt{1 - \sin^2\zeta}}} \leq \frac{12\, d\varepsilon}{|\sin\zeta|} \leq 12\, d\varepsilon^{2/3}.$$

Hence, for any $\beta \in N_0$ the projections $V_1(\beta)$ and $V_2''(\beta)$ are $24\, d\varepsilon^{2/3}$-proximate in the sense of ρ_h.

Since the set N_0 intersects all meridians in S^2 and for each unit vector $\omega \in S^2$ there exists a vector $\beta \in N_0$ orthogonal to ω, the convex bodies V_1 and V_2'' in R^3 are $24\, d\varepsilon^{2/3}$-proximate as well. Indeed, if some point $x \in \mathbb{R}^3$ is sufficiently far from a convex body V, i.e., $\rho_h(V, x) > \delta$, then there exists a vector $\omega \in N_0$ such that the analogous inequality $\rho_h(V(\omega), x(\omega)) > \delta$ holds on the plane $P(\omega)$ for the corresponding projections.

c. Now, let us suppose that the set N_0 does not contain the indicated triple of vectors $\beta_1, \beta_2, \beta_3$. Then it is contained in the $\varepsilon^{1/3}$-neighborhood of the great circle $C_0(\omega_0) \subset P(\omega_0)$, and we can assume that this circle contains the endpoints of two orthogonal vectors $\gamma_1, \gamma_2 \in N_0$. It is not difficult to verify that for all the vectors $\omega \in C_0(\omega_0)$ the ρ_t-distance between the projections $V_1(\omega)$ and $V_2(\omega)$ does not exceed $3\, d(\varepsilon + \varepsilon^{1/3})$.

c.1. If the set of angles $\{\Phi(\omega_0)\}$ contains an angle that is not greater than $\varepsilon^{2/3}$ in absolute value, then the translative distance between $V_1(\omega_0)$ and $V_2(\omega_0)$ does not exceed $3\, d(\varepsilon + \varepsilon^{2/3})$. Hence, Groemer's estimates imply that the ρ_t-distance between the bodies V_1 and V_2 in $\mathbb{R}^3$ does not exceed $3(1 + 2\sqrt{2})\, d(\varepsilon + \varepsilon^{2/3})$.

Note that, according to the previous lemma, any great circle, say $C(\omega_2)$, intersects the set N_0. Let $\omega_3 \in C(\omega_2) \cap N_0$. Since $V_1(\omega_3)$ and $V_2(\omega_3)$ are translationally $1.5\, d\varepsilon$-proximate, in any direction $\omega \perp \omega_3$, in particular, in the direction of ω_2, the widths of the bodies V_1 and V_2 satisfy the estimate $|H_1(\omega) - H_2(\omega)| < 3\, d\varepsilon$.

c.2. Now we consider the case when all the angles from the set $\{\Phi(\omega_0)\}$ are greater than $\varepsilon^{2/3}$ in absolute value.

Lemma 2.4.5. *If for the constructed unit normal vector $\omega_0 \perp C_0(\omega_0)$ all angles from the set $\Phi(\omega_0) \subset S^1$ are greater than $\varepsilon^{2/3}$, then the widths of the projections $V_1(\omega_0)$ and $V_2(\omega_0)$ are $12\pi\, d\varepsilon^{1/3}$-proximate to a constant.*

Proof. The width of V_1 in the direction of a unit vector γ_1 in the plane $P(\omega_0)$ is $1.5\, d\varepsilon$-proximate to the width of V_2 in the direction of γ_1 and $2\, d\varepsilon$-proximate to the widths of V_2 in the directions of the vectors $\{\gamma_1(\omega_0)\}$ that form angles from the segment $I(\omega_0, \varepsilon)$ with γ_1. Now we turn the plane $P(\omega_0)$ so that the normal vector ω of the rotating plane moves along the great circle that joins ω_0 with γ_2. Note that $\gamma_1 \perp \gamma_2$ by definition. In each of these planes $P(\omega)$ the width of V_1 satisfies the following estimates:

$$|H_1(\gamma_1) - H_2(\gamma_1)| < 2 \cdot 1.5\, d\varepsilon, \quad |H_1(\gamma_1) - H_2(\gamma_1(\omega))| < 2\, d\varepsilon$$

where $\gamma_1(\omega) \in C(\omega)$ is defined by analogy with the vectors $\gamma_1(\omega_0) \in C_0(\omega_0)$.

When the vector ω varies in the great circle $C(\gamma_1)$, the union of the sets of the vectors $\gamma_1(\omega)$ forms a neighborhood U of a certain closed curve s_1 which joins the endpoints of the vectors γ_1 and $\gamma_1(\omega_0)$ on the unit sphere and bounds some neighborhood of the minimal arc $(\gamma_1, \gamma_1(\omega_0))$.

We claim that the width of the body V_1 on this arc is almost constant. Let $\gamma_3 \in (\gamma_1, \gamma_1(\omega_0))$. Consider a closed curve s_3 which joins the endpoints of the vectors γ_3 and $\gamma_3(\omega_0)$ and is defined exactly as the curve s_1. Clearly, the intersection of the curves s_1 and s_3 is nonempty and the widths of V_1 and V_2 in the directions that belong to the intersection $s_1 \cap s_3$ are $3\, d\varepsilon$-proximate. Therefore,

$$|H_1(\gamma_1) - H_2(\gamma_3)| < 4 \cdot 1.5\, d\varepsilon$$

for any vector $\gamma_3 \in (\gamma_1, \gamma_1(\omega_0))$.

Since the ratio of the lengths of the circle $C_0(\omega_0)$ and the arc $(\gamma_1, \gamma_1(\omega_0))$ equals $2\pi\varepsilon^{-2/3}$, the width of the projection $V_1(\omega_0)$ is constant to within $4 \cdot 1.5\, d\varepsilon 2\pi/\varepsilon^{2/3} = 12\pi\, d\varepsilon^{1/3}$. □

The assertion of Theorem 2.4.1 for the case when all the projections of V_1 do not have constant width follows from the proximity of the widths of $V_1(\omega_0)$ to a constant.

Now we sum up our previous arguments.

a.1. If for any vector $\omega \in S^2$ the set of angles $\{\varphi(\omega)\}$ contains an angle less than $\varepsilon^{1/3}$, then the bodies V_1 and V_2 are translationally $(1 + 2\sqrt{2})(\varepsilon + \varepsilon^{1/3})\, d$-proximate.

a.2. If for any ω the set $\{\varphi(\omega)\}$ is contained in the $\varepsilon^{1/3}$-neighborhood of the angle $\pi \in S^1$, then the bodies V_1 and V_2 are centrally symmetric to each other with the same precision.

b. If for certain vectors ω the sets $\{\varphi(\omega)\}$ do not intersect the $\varepsilon^{1/3}$-neighborhoods of the points 0 and π of the unit circle and the above-mentioned set $N_0 \subset S^2$ (or N_π, as in Lemma 2.4.6) contains a triple of vectors $\beta_1, \beta_2, \beta_3$ such that $|\langle \beta_1, \beta_2, \beta_3 \rangle| > \varepsilon^{1/3}$, then the bodies V_1 and V_2 are congruent in $\mathbb{R}^3$ to within $24\, d\varepsilon^{2/3}$ with respect to some parallel translation or a central symmetry.

c.1. If the set N_0 (or N_π) *a priori* does not contain such a triple of vectors, and if $\{\Phi(\omega_0)\}$ contains an angle which is not greater than $\varepsilon^{2/3}$, then the bodies V_1 and V_2 are translationally $d(1 + 2\sqrt{2})3(\varepsilon + \varepsilon^{1/3})$-proximate.

c.2. If all the angles in the set $\{\Phi(\omega_0)\}$ are greater than $\varepsilon^{2/3}$, then the widths of the projections $V_1(\omega_0)$ and $V_2(\omega_0)$ are $12\pi\, d\varepsilon^{1/3}$-proximate to a constant.

Hence, Theorem 2.4.1 is proved in all possible cases. □

As was noted in Golubyatnikov (1982b), the limit of a sequence of 1-visible compact bodies in $\mathbb{R}^3$ may not be 1-visible, and the stability results for visible bodies are not true in general.

Consider a sufficiently dense spiral on the unit sphere $S^2 \subset \mathbb{R}^3$ going from one pole to the other. Using the "rectilinear knife", peel this spiral with some neighborhood from the unit ball $B \subset \mathbb{R}^3$, as one does when peeling potatoes. We can do this peeling in such a way that the line midway between two adjacent circuits of the spiral remains on the boundary ∂B with some neighborhood. Obviously, the part W which is cut away is a 1-visible body and the Hausdorff distance from W to the center of the ball B is almost one. However, any projection of B is sufficiently close in all possible senses to the corresponding projection of W.

Following the main ideas of the theory of ill-posed problems, we describe the class of visible compact bodies for which the stability of reconstruction of the form of a body from the forms of its projections can be established.

A compact body $W \subset \mathbb{R}^n$ is called *α-rough* if any point $x \notin W$ is contained in some dihedral angle of size α whose interior is disjoint from W. Here $0 < \alpha \leq \pi$.

For $\alpha = \pi$ we get the class of convex compact bodies.

For these α-rough objects the existence of stability similar to Theorem 2.4.1 can be obtained, but the exact estimates of this stability seem to be too hard to derive.

Chapter 3.

Other groups of congruences of projections

3.1. $SO(2)$-SIMILARITY OF PROJECTIONS

The notions of $SO(2)$-congruence and $SO(2)$-similarity of sets in Euclidean spaces do not seem to be principally different, and most results of the previous chapter can be extended to the group of $SO(2)$-similar projections of convex, $(n-2)$-convex and $(n-2)$-visible bodies in $\mathbb{R}^n$ onto two-dimensional planes.

Theorem 3.1.1. *Let $V_1, V_2 \subset \mathbb{R}^n$, $n \geq 3$, be compact convex bodies such that*

(1) their projections $V_1(P^2)$ and $V_2(P^2)$ onto any two-dimensional plane $P^2 \subset \mathbb{R}^n$ are $SO(2)$-similar (the ratio of the similitude is not supposed to be constant, independent of the plane P^2 !) and

(2) these projections have no $SO(2)$-symmetries.

Then the bodies V_1 and V_2 are either parallel or directly homothetic in $\mathbb{R}^n$.

In a natural way, the homothety with negative coefficient will be decomposed into the composition of a central symmetry and a homothety with positive coefficient.

Proof. Let us consider the case $n = 3$. The function $\varphi(\omega)$ defined as in Section 2.1 is continuous and it is easy to see that for all $\omega \in \varphi^{-1}(0) \cup \varphi^{-1}(\pi)$ the ratios of similitude of the projections $V_1(\omega)$ and $V_2(\omega)$ do not depend on ω. So, we can assume that they are equal to one. It is not difficult to verify that for any vector ω which is perpendicular to some $\omega_0 \in \varphi^{-1}(0) \cup \varphi^{-1}(\pi)$ the width functions w_1 and w_2 of the bodies V_1 and V_2 coincide: $w_1(\omega) = w_2(\omega)$.

Now, suppose that there exists a unit vector $\omega_1 \notin \varphi^{-1}(0) \cup \varphi^{-1}(\pi)$. As in Theorem 2.1.1, any vector $\omega_2 \in E(\omega_1)$ is perpendicular to some $\omega_3 \in \varphi^{-1}(0) \cup \varphi^{-1}(\pi)$, since the great circle $E(\omega_2)$ consists of two meridians with endpoints at $\pm\omega_1$. Each of these meridians intersect this union of the preimages.

Hence, the widths of the projections $V_1(\omega_1)$ and $V_2(\omega_1)$ coincide in all directions in the plane $P(\omega_1)$. The ratio of the similitude of these projections equals one because the maximum values of their width functions should be equal.

So, for all directions $\omega \in S^2$ the ratio of the similitude of the projections $V_1(\omega)$ and $V_2(\omega)$ equals one; therefore, these projections are $SO(2)$-congruent, and in the case $n = 3$ our theorem follows from Theorem 2.1.1. The case $n > 3$ can be treated by induction exactly as in Theorem 2.1.2. □

The results of Section 2.3 can be extended to the case of similar projections as well.

Theorem 3.1.2. *Let $W_1, W_2 \subset \mathbb{R}^n$, $n \geq 3$, be compact $(n-2)$-convex bodies such that*

(1) their projections $W_1(P^2)$ and $W_2(P^2)$ are $SO(2)$-similar for any two-dimensional plane $P^2 \subset \mathbb{R}^n$ (as above, the ratio of the similitude is not supposed to be constant, independent of the plane P^2) and

(2) the convex hulls of these projections have no $SO(2)$-symmetries.

Then W_1 and W_2 are either parallel or directly homothetic in $\mathbb{R}^n$.

Proof. Since the convex hulls $\operatorname{conv} W_1$ and $\operatorname{conv} W_2$ of the bodies W_1 and W_2 have $SO(2)$-similar projections onto any two-dimensional plane, it follows from Theorem 3.1.1, that these convex hulls are congruent with respect to either parallel translation T or to a homothety H. Suppose that this transformation $F = T$ or H is not a congruence of the bodies W_1 and W_2, say, $F(W_1) \neq W_2$, while $F(\operatorname{conv} W_1) = \operatorname{conv} W_2$, and that some point $M \in F(W_1)$ is not contained in W_2 (or vice versa). As in Theorem 2.3.1, consider an $(n-2)$-dimensional plane P containing this point M and disjoint from W_2. Let Q^2 be the orthogonal complement of P in $\mathbb{R}^n$. The projections of the $(n-2)$-convex bodies $F(W_1)$ and W_2 onto Q^2 are $SO(2)$-congruent and the convex hulls of these projections coincide. Therefore, the projection of $F(W_1)$ onto Q^2 can be obtained from the corresponding projection of W_2 neither by a nonzero translation nor by a rotation, since the convex hulls of these projections have no $SO(2)$-symmetries. This contradicts the existence of the point M. □

Theorem 3.1.3. *Let $W_1, W_2 \subset \mathbb{R}^n$, $n \geq 3$, be compact $(n-2)$-visible simply connected bodies such that*

(1) their projections $W_1(P^2)$ and $W_2(P^2)$ are $SO(2)$-similar for any two-dimensional plane $P^2 \subset \mathbb{R}^n$ (as above, the ratio of the similitude is not supposed to be constant, independent of the plane P^2) and

(2) these projections have no $SO(2)$-symmetries.

Then W_1 and W_2 are either parallel or directly homothetic in $\mathbb{R}^n$.

The proof of this theorem repeats the corresponding arguments of Theorems 3.1.1 and 2.3.2.

We have already mentioned in Section 2.3 that the absence of $SO(2)$-symmetries of the projections in the case of $(n-2)$-convex and $(n-2)$-visible bodies is essential for the uniqueness of reconstruction of the shapes of these bodies, and it was not difficult to construct the corresponding counterexamples. It is amazing that for the group of similarity transformations of the projections this asymmetry is essential in the case of convex bodies as well. Namely, in Theorem 3.1.1 the condition of the absence of symmetries of the projections cannot be removed, as was shown by the following examples constructed in Petty and McKinney (1987).

Let $V_1, V_2 \subset \mathbb{R}^n$, $n \geq 3$, be compact centrally symmetric bodies with support functions

$$h_1(x) = |x| \cdot \exp\Big(\frac{\langle Ax, x\rangle}{|x|^2}\Big),$$
$$h_2(x) = |x| \cdot \exp\Big(-\frac{\langle Ax, x\rangle}{|x|^2}\Big). \tag{3.1.1}$$

Here $x \in \mathbb{R}^n$, $|x|$ is the norm of this vector, and A is a symmetric $n \times n$ matrix whose eigenvalues $\lambda_1, \dots, \lambda_n$ satisfy the condition

$$\max |\lambda_i - \lambda_j| \leq 1/2. \tag{3.1.2}$$

This inequality provides the positivity of the curvature radius of the boundary of the projection $\dfrac{d^2h}{d\varphi^2} + h$ for all directions tangent to the unit sphere for both support functions h_1 and h_2, which implies the convexity of these bodies V_1 and V_2 (see, for example, Pogorelov, 1973).

Direct computations show that the projections of these bodies onto two-dimensional plane $P(u, v)$ spanned on the orthogonal pair of unit vectors $u, v \in S^{n-1}$ are similar with the ratio of the similitude $\exp(\langle Av, v\rangle + \langle Au, u\rangle)$, and after rotation by the angle $\pi/2$ these projections become directly homothetic. We shall reproduce similar computations below in the case of convex bodies in complex Euclidean spaces. For a wide class of matrices A, these convex bodies $V_1, V_2 \subset \mathbb{R}^n$ are not affinely equivalent. The explicit description of such matrices was given by Gardner and Volčič (1994) (see also Gardner, 1995) in the following theorem:

Theorem. *The convex bodies V_1 and V_2 of the Petty-McKinney example are affinely equivalent if and only if they are similar, and this occurs if and only if there is a constant a such that the eigenvalues λ_i of the matrix A arranged so that they increase with i satisfy the relations*

$$\lambda_i + \lambda_{n+1-i} = a, \qquad i = 1, \dots, n. \tag{3.1.3}$$

In particular, the diagonal matrix with eigenvalues

$$\lambda_1 = 1/2, \qquad \lambda_i = 1, \qquad i = 2, 3, \dots, n \tag{3.1.4}$$

belongs to this class.

Gardner and Volčič have also indicated there that if this condition is satisfied and the matrix A is not a scalar one ($A \neq \lambda E$, where E is the unit matrix), then these bodies V_1 and V_2 are similar but not directly homothetic.

Analogous example in the case of complex Euclidean spaces was constructed by N. Baltakhinova and the author.

Let $\mathcal{V}_1, \mathcal{V}_2 \subset \mathbb{C}^n$, $n \geq 3$, be compact centrally symmetric bodies with support functions

$$h_1(x) = |x|_{\mathbb{C}} \cdot \exp\Big(\frac{\langle Ax, x\rangle_{\mathbb{C}}}{|x|^2_{\mathbb{C}}}\Big),$$
$$h_2(x) = |x|_{\mathbb{C}} \cdot \exp\Big(-\frac{\langle Ax, x\rangle_{\mathbb{C}}}{|x|^2_{\mathbb{C}}}\Big). \tag{3.1.5}$$

Here $x \in \mathbb{C}^n$, $\langle \cdot, \cdot \rangle_{\mathbb{C}}$ denotes the Hermitian scalar product in $\mathbb{C}^n$, $|x|^2_{\mathbb{C}} = \langle x, x\rangle_{\mathbb{C}}$ is the corresponding norm of this vector, and A is a Hermitian $n \times n$ complex matrix whose eigenvalues $\lambda_1, \dots, \lambda_n$ satisfy the condition (3.1.2). Obviously, the scalar product $\langle Ax, x\rangle_{\mathbb{C}}$ is real for any vector $x \in \mathbb{C}^n$.

The natural correspondence

$$x + \mathrm{i}y \longleftrightarrow \begin{pmatrix} x & y \\ -y & x \end{pmatrix}$$

which identifies the complex Euclidean space $\mathbb{C}^n$ with the real space $\mathbb{R}^{2n}$ transforms the complex Hermitian $n \times n$ matrix A into the real symmetric $2n \times 2n$ matrix $\mathcal{A}$. Clearly, the eigenvalues $\lambda_1, \lambda_1, \lambda_2, \lambda_2, \dots, \lambda_n, \lambda_n$ of $\mathcal{A}$ satisfy the condition (3.1.2) as well.

According to Petty and McKinney (1987), the bodies $\mathcal{V}_1, \mathcal{V}_2 \subset \mathbb{R}^{2n}$ are convex and their projections onto any two-dimensional **real** plane are $SO(2)$-similar and after rotation of one of them by the angle $\pi/2$ about the origin they become directly homothetic in this plane.

The theorem of Gardner and Volčič mentioned above shows that these convex bodies $\mathcal{V}_1$ and $\mathcal{V}_2$ are affinely equivalent if and only if they are similar themselves, and this is so if and only if the condition (3.1.3) is satisfied for the eigenvalues of the matrix A. It is obvious that in this case the eigenvalues of the matrix $\mathcal{A}$ also satisfy the condition (3.1.3).

Now, consider the projections of the bodies $\mathcal{V}_1$ and $\mathcal{V}_2$ onto any two-dimensional *complex* plane $P^2_{\mathbb{C}} \subset \mathbb{C}^n$. Actually, we shall follow the idea of the corresponding construction in $\mathbb{R}^n$ described in Gardner (1995).

By the definition of the support functions, the orthogonal projection of a convex body V onto any plane P is described by the restriction of the support function of V to the plane P. Let $\{u, v\}$ be any orthonormal basis in the plane $P^2_{\mathbb{C}}$ (in the sense of the Hermitian scalar product). For any unit vector $z = (z_1, z_2) = z_1 \cdot u + z_2 \cdot v$ in this plane, we have

$$\begin{aligned} \ln(h_1(z)) &= \langle A(z_1 \cdot u + z_2 \cdot v), z_1 \cdot u + z_2 \cdot v \rangle_{\mathbb{C}} \\ &= \langle Au, u \rangle_{\mathbb{C}} \cdot |z_1|^2 + \langle Au, v \rangle_{\mathbb{C}} \cdot z_1 \overline{z}_2 \\ &\quad + \langle Av, u \rangle_{\mathbb{C}} \cdot \overline{z}_1 z_2 + \langle Av, v \rangle_{\mathbb{C}} \cdot |z_2|^2 . \end{aligned}$$

Let $\tilde{z} = (-\overline{z}_2, \overline{z}_1) = -\overline{z}_2 \cdot u + \overline{z}_1 \cdot v$. Then

$$\begin{aligned} \ln(h_2(\tilde{z})) &= \langle -A(-\overline{z}_2 \cdot u + \overline{z}_1 \cdot v), -\overline{z}_2 \cdot u + \overline{z}_1 \cdot v \rangle_{\mathbb{C}} \\ &= -\langle Au, u \rangle_{\mathbb{C}} \cdot |z_2|^2 + \langle Au, v \rangle_{\mathbb{C}} \cdot z_1 \overline{z}_2 \\ &\quad + \langle Av, u \rangle_{\mathbb{C}} \cdot \overline{z}_1 z_2 - \langle Av, v \rangle_{\mathbb{C}} \cdot |z_1|^2 . \end{aligned}$$

Since the vector z has unit length, we have $|z_1|^2 + |z_2|^2 = 1$ and thus

$$\frac{h_1(z)}{h_2(\tilde{z})} = \exp\left(\langle Au, u \rangle_{\mathbb{C}} + \langle Av, v \rangle_{\mathbb{C}}\right) = K(P^2_{\mathbb{C}}).$$

This is a real number which does not depend on the choice of the vector $z \in P^2_{\mathbb{C}}$. Hence, the projection of the body $\mathcal{V}_1$ onto the plane $P^2_{\mathbb{C}}$ and the image of the corresponding projection of the body $\mathcal{V}_2$ under the linear inversely conformal transformation

$$S : (z_1, z_2) \longrightarrow (-\overline{z}_2, \overline{z}_1)$$

of this plane are directly homothetic with the coefficient $K(P^2_{\mathbb{C}})$.

Note that, exactly as in the case of the real Euclidean spaces, this transformation S can be interpreted as the rotation by the angle $\pi/2$, since the vectors (z_1, z_2) and $(-\overline{z}_2, \overline{z}_1)$ are perpendicular in the sense of the Hermitian scalar product.

As we have seen in Section 2.1, the rotation function $\varphi : S^2 \longrightarrow S^1$ cannot be well defined for the pairs of convex bodies in $\mathbb{R}^3$ whose projections onto some two-dimensional planes have $SO(2)$-symmetries. If these bodies are centrally symmetric, then the order of symmetry of their projections is even, and one can hope to define another rotation function $\tilde{\varphi} : S^2 \longrightarrow S^1$, say $\tilde{\varphi}(\omega) = 2 \cdot \varphi(\omega)$, in order to reproduce the proof of Theorem 3.1.1 for the centrally symmetric bodies.

For the particular case (3.1.4) of the diagonal matrix A with $\lambda_1 = 1/2$, $\lambda_2 = \lambda_3 = 1$, the projections of the convex bodies $V_1, V_2 \subset \mathbb{R}^3$ onto the plane $x^1 = 0$ are circular, and in this case it is impossible to define the rotation function φ for the vector $\omega = (1, 0, 0)$ correctly. Nevertheless, there is still a hope that for the symmetric 3×3 matrices without multiple eigenvalues, $\lambda_1 \neq \lambda_2 \neq \lambda_3 \neq \lambda_1$, such a modified rotation function can be defined.

Suppose that for some matrix A as above the restriction of the quadratic form $\langle Ax, x\rangle$ on any plane $P(\omega) \subset \mathbb{R}^3$ has different eigenvalues $\Lambda_1(\omega) > \Lambda_2(\omega)$. This assumption is equivalent to the nonexistence of circular projections of the bodies V_1 and V_2. The directions of the eigenvector corresponding to the largest eigenvalue $\Lambda_1(\omega)$ determine a continuous field of tangent directions in the tangent space TS^2 of the unit sphere. It is well known that such fields do not exist on even-dimensional spheres.

Hence, for any pair of convex bodies $V_1, V_2 \subset \mathbb{R}^3$ from the Petty–McKinney example (3.1.1), there exists at least one pair of unit vectors $\pm\omega_0 \in S^2$ such that the projections of the bodies V_1 and V_2 onto the plane $P(\omega_0)$ are circular. So, the rotation function φ cannot be modified for any example of this kind.

The following natural question was formulated in Gardner and Volčič (1994):

Question. *Suppose V_1 and V_2 are centrally symmetric convex bodies in E^n such that $V_1(P^2)$ is similar to $V_2(P^2)$ for every two-dimensional plane P^2. Must V_1 and V_2 be a pair as in the Petty–McKinney example?*

Similar results for the sections of convex bodies can be obtained using the polar duality construction. In particular, the proof of the next theorem follows the scheme of that of Theorem 2.1.3.

Theorem 3.1.4. *Let $V_1, V_2 \subset \mathbb{R}^n$, $n \geq 3$, be compact convex bodies and $q_i \in V_i$, $i = 1, 2$, be their interior points. If the sections of these bodies given by parallel two-dimensional planes containing q_1 and q_2 are $SO(2)$-similar and have no $SO(2)$-symmetries and the points q_1 and q_2 correspond to each other in these similarities, then the bodies V_1 and V_2 are either parallel in $\mathbb{R}^n$ or directly homothetic (possibly with negative homothety coefficient).*

The Petty–McKinney examples show that the condition of the absence of symmetries of the sections in this theorem is essential as well.

3.2. $SO(3)$-CONGRUENCE OF PROJECTIONS

In this section we consider our Main Question in the case when two convex or visible bodies have the same shapes of their projections onto three-dimensional planes in a real Euclidean space.

Theorem 3.2.1. *Let V_1 and V_2 be compact convex bodies in $\mathbb{R}^n$, $n \geq 4$, for which*

(1) the width functions have finitely many maxima;

(2) for any three-dimensional plane $P^3 \subset \mathbb{R}^n$ their projections $V_1(P^3)$ and $V_2(P^3)$ onto this plane are $SO(3)$-congruent and have no $SO(3)$-symmetries.

Then V_1 and V_2 are parallel in $\mathbb{R}^n$.

Note that as in the previous chapter, the class of all convex compact sets in $\mathbb{R}^n$ which satisfy the assumptions of this theorem constitute an open everywhere dense set in the sense of the Hausdorff metric.

The difference of the statements of this theorem and its two-dimensional analogue, Theorem 2.1.2, is based on the orientation properties of the antipodal maps $x \longleftrightarrow -x$ in $\mathbb{R}^n$. In the case of even-dimensional spaces they do not change the orientations and in odd-dimensional spaces they do not preserve it. Thus, taking instead of one of the bodies V_i the corresponding $\widehat{V}_i$ which is centrally symmetric to V_i, we obtain a simple corollary of Theorem 3.2.1:

Theorem 3.2.2. *Let V_1 and V_2 be convex compact bodies in $\mathbb{R}^n$, $n \geq 4$, and assume that*

(1) their width functions have finitely many maxima;

(2) for any three-dimensional plane $P^3 \subset \mathbb{R}^n$, their projections $V_1(P^3)$ and $V_2(P^3)$ are unorientably congruent and have no $SO(3)$-symmetries.

Then V_1 is centrally symmetric to V_2 in $\mathbb{R}^n$.

Proof of Theorem 3.2.1 is based on consideration of the case $n = 4$. If the projections of V_1 and V_2 onto any four-dimensional plane in $\mathbb{R}^n$ are parallel, then, according to Süss's lemma, the same is true for their projections onto any five-dimensional plane and the general case follows from Süss's lemma by induction.

The following lemmas will be needed in the sequel:

Lemma 3.2.1. *Let G be a compact set of affine transformations in $\mathbb{R}^n$ and let $V_1, V_2 \subset \mathbb{R}^n$ be compact convex bodies such that*

(1) for any ω, the projection $V_1(\omega)$ onto a hyperplane $P(\omega)$ is transformed into the corresponding projection $V_2(\omega)$ by some $\Phi(\omega) \in G$ which does not change the direction and the length of ω;

(2) all these projections have no symmetries with respect to such transformations from the group G.

Then $\Phi(\omega)$ is uniquely determined and depends on ω continuously.

Proof. The first part of the statement is obvious. Suppose that the mapping $\Phi : S^{n-1} \longrightarrow G$ has a discontinuity point ω_* and choose two sequences of unit vectors ψ_i and χ_i convergent to ω_* which have different limits of $\Phi(\psi_i)$ and $\Phi(\chi_i)$. These limits do exist because of the compactness of G. Hence, the projection $V_1(\omega_*)$ can be transformed into $V_2(\omega_*)$ by different transformations from G and this contradicts to the assumption that the projections of V_1 and V_2 have no G-symmetries. □

Similar continuity property was established in Section 2.1 for the rotation angle mapping $\varphi : S^2 \longrightarrow S^1$ in the case of projections onto two-dimensional planes.

Lemma 3.2.2. *If $V_1, V_2 \subset \mathbb{R}^3$ are compact convex bodies and their projections onto any plane have no axes of symmetry, then for some $\omega \in S^2$ the projections $V_1(\omega)$ and $V_2(\omega)$ are not unorientably $O(2)$-congruent.*

Proof. Suppose that for all $\omega \in S^2$ the projections $V_1(\omega)$ and $V_2(\omega)$ are unorientably $O(2)$-congruent.

Any isometry of a plane $P(\omega)$ that does not preserve the orientation can be represented as a composition of a symmetry with respect to some axis $l(\omega)$ and a parallel translation along $l(\omega)$. It follows from the asymmetry of $V_1(\omega)$ and $V_2(\omega)$ that for any $\omega \in S^2$ the direction of the axis $l(\omega)$ is well defined, and, according to Lemma 3.2.1, this direction depends on ω continuously, but neither the sphere S^2 nor the projective plane RP^2 have continuous fields of directions in their tangent bundles, which contradicts the assumption on congruence above. □

Lemma 3.2.3. *Let $V_1, V_2 \subset \mathbb{R}^n$, $n \geq 4$, be convex compact bodies and assume that their projections onto any 3-dimensional plane are $O(3)$-congruent. Then the width functions $w_1(\omega)$ and $w_2(\omega)$ of these bodies coincide for all $\omega \in S^{n-1}$.*

Proof. Clearly, it is sufficient to consider the case $n = 4$. Let $\overline{V}_1$ and $\overline{V}_2$ be convex bodies in $\mathbb{R}^4$ obtained from V_1 and V_2, respectively, by the symmetrization with respect to the origin. It is well-known that the support functions of these origin-symmetric bodies $\overline{V}_i$, $i = 1, 2$, satisfy the following identities:

$$\overline{h}_i(\omega) = \overline{h}_i(-\omega) = \frac{h_i(\omega) + h_i(-\omega)}{2} = \frac{w_i(\omega)}{2}. \tag{3.2.1}$$

Since the projections $V_1(\omega)$ and $V_2(\omega)$ onto any hyperplane $P^3(\omega) \subset \mathbb{R}^4$ are $O(3)$-congruent, the same is true for the corresponding projections $\overline{V}_1(\omega)$ and $\overline{V}_2(\omega)$. Thus, the spherical Radon transform of the even support functions $\overline{h}_1(\omega)$ and $\overline{h}_2(\omega)$ coincide for any hyperplane:

$$R\overline{h}_1(\omega) = R\overline{h}_2(\omega) = \int\limits_{S^2(\omega)} \overline{h}_1(m)\,\mathrm{d}m = \int\limits_{S^2(\omega)} \overline{h}_2(\omega)\,\mathrm{d}m. \tag{3.2.2}$$

Here $S^2(\omega) = S^3 \cap P^3(\omega)$ is a unit sphere in the hyperplane $P^3(\omega)$. As was shown in Helgason (1984), there is an explicit inversion formula for the spherical Radon transform on S^3:

$$R^{-1}\overline{h} = \frac{1}{16\pi^2} \cdot R(1 - \Delta)\overline{h},$$

where Δ is the Laplacian on the unit sphere S^3. These inversions of the spherical Radon transform were used by Gardner, Koldobsky and Schlumprecht (1999) in their solution to the Busemann-Petty problem.

The integral equation (3.2.2) has a unique solution in the class of even functions on this sphere: $\overline{h}_1(\omega) = \overline{h}_2(\omega) = \overline{h}(\omega)$, and it follows from (3.2.1) that $w_1(\omega) = w_2(\omega)$. □

In particular, this uniqueness implies that convex centrally symmetric compact bodies with $O(3)$-congruent projections onto any 3-dimensional plane in $\mathbb{R}^n$, $n \geq 4$, are parallel.

Proof of Theorem 3.2.1. We begin the proof of Theorem 3.2.1 from the case when $V_1, V_2 \subset \mathbb{R}^4$ and their width functions $h_1(\omega) = h_2(\omega)$ have maximum on the unique pair of the unit vectors $\pm p$. We can assume that one of these bodies is moved by a parallel translation in a position such that the boundary points $x^+, x^- \in V_1$ and $y^+, y^- \in V_2$ with outward normals $\pm p$ to the corresponding support planes coincide pairwise.

For any $\omega \in S^2(p) \subset P(p)$, the projections $V_1(\omega)$ and $V_2(\omega) \subset P(\omega)$ can be transformed into each other

(1) by the identical isometry;

(2) or by a rotation about the straight line P parallel to p and containing the points x^+, x^-;

(3) or by the rotation through the angle π about an axis $A(\omega)$ orthogonal to p.

Let us denote the corresponding sets of all such vectors ω by S_1, S_2 and S_3, respectively. All these subsets of $S^2(p)$ are centrally symmetric. Since the projections $V_i(\omega)$ have no $SO(3)$-symmetries, the sets S_1 and S_3 are closed and do not intersect each other. It is easy to see that the set S_3 does not intersect the closure of S_2, though S_1 can do it.

Hence, either the projections $V_1(\omega)$ and $V_2(\omega)$ are congruent with respect to the rotations through the angle π about the axis $A(\omega)$ for all $\omega \in S^2(p)$ or these projections are congruent with respect to some rotations through the angle $\varphi(\omega)$ (possibly equal to zero) about the line l. According to Lemma 3.2.1, this angle of rotation depends on ω continuously because the projections of the bodies V_1 and V_2 have no SO-symmetries. In the first of these two mutually exclusive cases, as in Lemma 3.2.2, we obtain a continuous field of tangent directions on the sphere $S^2(p)$, which is impossible. Therefore, we have to study only the second case.

Let $\varphi : S^2(p) \to S^1$ be the continuous map as above.

Given any $\omega \in S^2(p)$, consider the positively oriented orthonormal basis (p, ω, e_1, e_2) in $\mathbb{R}^4$. The projection $V_1(\omega)$ is transformed into $V_2(\omega)$ by some rotation in the plane of the vectors e_1 and e_2 through the angle $\varphi(\omega)$. Since the positively oriented orthonormal basis $(p, -\omega, \varepsilon_1, \varepsilon_2)$ has opposite orientation in the plane of the pair ε_1 , ε_2 with respect to that of the pair e_1, e_2, we have

$$\varphi(-\omega) = -\varphi(\omega).$$

It can be verified as in Section 2.1 that if for some $\omega_0 \in S^2(p)$ $\pi \neq \varphi(\omega_0) \neq 0$, then all the meridians of $S^2(p)$ with ends at the points $\pm\omega_0$ do intersect the preimage $\varphi^{-1}(0)$ or the preimage $\varphi^{-1}(\pi)$. Note that both of these preimages are closed and centrally symmetric and the projections of V_1 and V_2 onto the planes orthogonal to the vectors from $\varphi^{-1}(0)$ coincide because $x^+ = y^+$ and $x^- = y^-$.

First, consider the case when all these meridians intersect $\varphi^{-1}(0)$. This means that for any $\omega \in S^3 \subset \mathbb{R}^4$ there exists some vector in $\varphi^{-1}(0)$ orthogonal to ω, and as far the projections of V_1 and V_2 onto the planes orthogonal to the vectors from this preimage coincide, the support functions of these bodies coincide identically, and in this case Theorem 3.2.1 is proved.

If all these meridians intersect $\varphi^{-1}(\pi)$, we take the convex compact body Λ_1 obtained from V_1 by the axial symmetry with respect to the straight line l. In this case, for any $\omega \in S^2(p)$, the projections $\Lambda_1(\omega)$, $V_2(\omega)$ determine a continuous map $\psi : S^2(p) \longrightarrow S^1$ such that the preimage $\psi^{-1}(0)$ intersects all the meridians of $S^2(p)$ with endpoints at $\pm\omega_0$. As above, we see that the bodies V_2 and Λ_1 coincide, but on the other hand, the projections $V_2(p)$ and $\Lambda_1(p)$ are centrally symmetric to each other by the construction, which means that both of these projections have centers of symmetry. This contradicts the assumptions of the theorem.

Now, suppose that the width functions of the bodies V_1 and V_2 have maximums at a finite set of directions $\pm p_1, \pm p_2, \dots \pm p_k$, $k > 1$.

Since the projections of the bodies V_1 and V_2 onto any hyperplane have no symmetries, the variations of the vector ω in the planes $P(p_i)$ show that if ω is orthogonal to some pair of directions $\pm p_\alpha$ and $\pm p_\beta$, then the corresponding projections $V_1(\omega)$ and $V_2(\omega)$ should be parallel. As in the case $k = 1$ above, every meridian of any sphere $S^2(p_i)$ intersects the preimage $\varphi^{-1}(0)$. Thus, for any $\omega \in S^2(p_i)$ the projections $V_1(\omega)$ and $V_2(\omega)$ are parallel, and our theorem follows from Süss's lemma. □

Theorems 3.2.1 and 3.2.2 are valid for some wider classes of nonconvex compact sets analogous to those considered in Section 2.3.

Theorem 3.2.3. *Let $W_1, W_2 \subset \mathbb{R}^n$, $n \geq 4$, be compact $(n-3)$-convex bodies. If the width functions of their convex hulls have finite sets of maximums, the projections of W_1 and W_2 onto any 3-dimensional plane in $\mathbb{R}^n$ are $SO(3)$-congruent and the convex hulls of these projections have no $SO(3)$-symmetries, then the bodies W_1 and W_2 are parallel in $\mathbb{R}^3$.*

Proof. The proof follows from Theorem 3.2.1, which asserts that the convex hulls of W_1 and W_2 are parallel in $\mathbb{R}^n$. If W_1 does not coincide with W_2 after this translation, then the convex hulls of some projections of these compact bodies would have rotation symmetries, which this contradicts the assumptions of the theorem. □

A similar result holds for the $(n-3)$-visible bodies in $\mathbb{R}^n$, since the projections of an $(n-3)$-visible compact in $\mathbb{R}^n$ onto any 4-dimensional plane are 1-visible (and 1-convex).

All results above can be generalized to wider classes of $SO(3)$-similar projections of compact bodies. Analogous transformations were considered in the previous section.

Theorem 3.2.4. *Let $W_1, W_2 \subset \mathbb{R}^n$, $n > 3$, be compact $(n-3)$-convex bodies and let their width functions have finite sets of maximums. Let their projections onto any 3-dimensional plane $P^3 \subset \mathbb{R}^n$ be $SO(3)$-similar and the convex hulls of these projections have no $SO(3)$-symmetries. (As in the previous section, we do not assume that the ratio of the similitude of these projections does not depend on the plane P^3). Then W_1 and W_2 are either parallel or directly homothetic with positive coefficient.*

This theorem can be reduced to the previous one using some homothety with coefficient equal to the ratio of the diameters of W_1 and W_2.

Similar statements about unorientably congruent projections are valid as well. In this case the initial compact bodies are transformed into each other in $\mathbb{R}^n$ by some direct homothety with negative coefficient.

3.3. $SU(2)$ AND U-CONGRUENCE OF PROJECTIONS

In this section we consider the orthogonal projections of compact convex bodies in the complex vector space onto two-dimensional complex planes. First, for simplicity, we take the group $SU(2)$ as the group of transformations of these projections.

We remind that two sets A_1 and A_2 in the complex two-dimensional space are called $SU(2)$-congruent if for some element $g \in SU(2)$ the sets $g(A_2)$ and A_1 are parallel in $\mathbb{C}^2$.

Theorem 3.3.1. *Let V_1 and V_2 be compact convex bodies in $\mathbb{C}^3$ such that*

(1) their projections $V_1(\omega)$ and $V_2(\omega)$ onto any two-dimensional complex plane $P(\omega) \subset \mathbb{C}^3$ are $SU(2)$-congruent and have no $SU(2)$-symmetries,

(2) for each of these bodies, its projections onto different complex lines are pairwise noncongruent with respect to the group $U(1)$ and have no $U(1)$-symmetries.

Then the bodies V_1 and V_2 are either parallel in $\mathbb{C}^3$ or centrally symmetric to each other.

The statement of the theorem means that for any vector $\omega \in S^5$ the transformation $\varphi(\omega) \in SU(2)$ of the projection $V_1(\omega)$ to $V_2(\omega)$ is described by a matrix $\pm E$, where E is the unit 2×2 matrix.

Proof. Suppose that for some $\omega_0 \in S^5$ the transformation $\varphi(\omega_0)$ does not have the form $\pm E$. Then in some orthonormal basis $\{e_1(\omega_0), e_2(\omega_0)\}$ of the plane $P(\omega_0)$ this transformation is described by the matrix

$$M_0 = \begin{pmatrix} \exp(\mathrm{i}\mu(\omega_0)) & 0 \\ 0 & \exp(-\mathrm{i}\mu(\omega_0)) \end{pmatrix},$$

where $\mu(\omega_0) \neq k\pi$ for integer k.

The projections of the bodies V_1 and V_2 onto the complex coordinate axis directed along the vector $e_1(\omega_0)$ are congruent with respect to multiplication by $\exp(\mathrm{i}\mu(\omega_0))$, and their projections onto the axis $Oe_2(\omega_0)$ are congruent with respect to multiplication by $\exp(-\mathrm{i}\mu(\omega_0))$.

We shall examine a little bit more general situation which will be useful in the sequel. Let l be a complex line in $\mathbb{C}^3$ parallel to a unit vector e and $\omega_1, \omega_2 \in P(e)$ be unit vectors orthogonal to e. Consider the planes $P(\omega_1)$ and $P(\omega_2)$ and the orthonormal bases $\{e_1(\omega_1), e\}$ and $\{e_1(\omega_2), e\}$, respectively, in these planes. Here the unit vectors $e_1(\omega_1) \in P(\omega_1)$ and $e_1(\omega_2) \in P(\omega_2)$ are determined uniquely up to the action of the group $U(1)$.

Lemma 3.3.1. *Let V_1 and V_2 be compact convex bodies in $\mathbb{C}^3$ such that*

(1) their projections $V_1(\omega)$ and $V_2(\omega)$ onto any two-dimensional complex plane $P(\omega) \subset \mathbb{C}^3$ are $U(2)$-congruent and have no $U(2)$-symmetries,

(2) for each of these bodies, its projections onto different complex lines are pairwise noncongruent with respect to the group $U(1)$ and have no $U(1)$-symmetries.

If the projections of the bodies V_1 and V_2 onto the line l are $U(1)$-congruent, then the matrices $M(\omega_1)$ and $M(\omega_2)$ of the $U(2)$-transformations $\varphi(\omega_1)$ and $\varphi(\omega_2)$, respectively, are diagonal in the bases $\{e_1(\omega_1), e\}$ and $\{e_1(\omega_2), e\}$, respectively, and their second eigenvalues coincide.

Proof. Consider the plane $P(\omega_1)$ and the basis $\{e_1(\omega_1), e\}$ in it. If the unitary matrix $M(\omega_1)$ is not diagonal in this basis, then the line l_1 which is parallel to the vector $\varphi(\omega_1)e$ is not parallel to the line l. The projections of the bodies V_1 and V_2 onto the line l are $U(1)$-congruent and their projections onto the plane $P(\omega_1)$ are $U(2)$-congruent:

$$\varphi(\omega_1) : V_2(\omega_1) \longrightarrow V_1(\omega_1).$$

Hence, the projections of the body V_1 onto the different lines l and l_1 are $U(1)$-congruent. We have $V_1(l) \sim V_2(l) \sim V_1(\varphi(\omega_1)l)$, which contradicts condition (2) of the lemma. The case of the matrix $M(\omega_2)$ is studied in the same way. □

Let $m(\omega_0, e_1)$ be the great circle on the sphere S^5 that contains the endpoints of the vectors ω_0 and $e_1(\omega_0)$ and let $\omega_1 \in S^5$ be any unit vector with endpoint on this circle. The axis $Oe_2(\omega_0)$ is perpendicular to any such vector ω_1 and, by virtue of condition (2), the projections of the bodies $V_1(\omega_1)$ and $V_2(\omega_1)$ lie in the plane $P(\omega_1)$ so that their projections onto the line $Oe_2(\omega_0)$ are congruent with respect to multiplication by $\exp(i\mu(\omega_0))$.

Hence, for any vector ω_1 with endpoint on the circle $m(\omega_0, e_1)$ the transformation $\varphi(\omega_1)$ is described by the diagonal matrix $M_0 \in SU(2)$ in the orthonormal basis $\{e_1(\omega_1), e_2(\omega_0)\}$ of the plane $P(\omega_1)$. Similarly, it can be verified that for any vector ω_2 which corresponds to the points of the great circle $m(\omega_0, e_2)$, defined exactly as $m(\omega_0, e_1)$, the transformation $\varphi(\omega_2)$ is described by the same matrix M_0.

Taking for the initial vector ω_0 any vector orthogonal to $e_2(\omega_0)$ or $e_1(\omega_0)$, one can verify using Lemma 3.3.1 that for any unit vector $\omega \in S^5$ the transformation $\varphi(\omega)$ is described by the matrix M_0 in some basis $\{e_1(\omega), e_2(\omega)\}$ of the plane $P(\omega)$.

The orbit of the action of the group $U(1)$ on the vector $\omega \in S^5$ obviously consists of the vectors orthogonal to the plane $P(\omega)$. Therefore, the representation $\varphi(\omega) \equiv M_0 = \text{const}$ allows us to decompose the orthogonal complement to these orbits on S^5 into the sum of two one-dimensional complex vector bundles corresponding to the vectors $e_1(\omega)$ and $e_2(\omega)$, which form a basis in the plane $P(\omega)$, and we obtain the following splitting of the tangent bundle of the sphere S^5:

$$TS^5 = \theta^1_R \oplus \eta^1_{\mathbb{C}}(e_1) \oplus \eta^1_{\mathbb{C}}(e_2), \tag{3.3.1}$$

where θ^1_R is the trivial one-dimensional real vector bundle tangent to the $U(1)$-orbits on S^5 and the one-dimensional complex vector bundles $\eta^1_{\mathbb{C}}(e_1)$, $\eta^1_{\mathbb{C}}(e_2)$ were indicated above.

As is well known, any two-dimensional real vector bundle on a sphere of dimension greater than 2 is trivial by virtue of the triviality of the homotopy groups

$$\pi_{k-1}(S^1) = \pi_{k-1}(SO(2)) = \pi_{k-1}(U(1))$$

for $k > 2$. Hence, the complex line bundles $\eta^1_{\mathbb{C}}(e_1)$ and $\eta^1_{\mathbb{C}}(e_2)$ are trivial as well. On the other hand, as was shown in Adams (1962), there are no two linearly independent vector fields on the five-dimensional sphere; therefore, the sum $\eta^1_{\mathbb{C}}(e_1) \oplus \eta^1_{\mathbb{C}}(e_2)$ cannot contain a trivial subbundle.

This contradicts the triviality of the vector bundles $\eta^1_{\mathbb{C}}(e_1)$ and $\eta^1_{\mathbb{C}}(e_2)$, which were constructed under the assumption that $\varphi(\omega_0) \neq \pm E$ for some unit vector ω_0, and this implies the assertion of our theorem. □

We have noted in Sections 2.1 and 3.1 that for the pairs of convex bodies in the three-dimensional space the rotation function can be well defined only if the projections of these bodies onto two-dimensional planes do not have $SO(2)$-symmetries. Similar phenomena appear in complex Euclidean spaces. Let $V_1, V_2 \subset \mathbb{C}^3$ be a pair of centrally symmetric convex bodies in the complex variant of Petty-McKinney's example defined by (3.1.5). Assume that for all unit vectors $\omega \in S^5$ the restrictions of the quadratic form $\langle Ax, x\rangle_{\mathbb{C}}$ to the complex plane $P^2_{\mathbb{C}}(\omega)$ have different eigenvalues: $\Lambda_1(\omega) > \Lambda_2(\omega)$. Since A is a Hermitian matrix, these eigenvalues are real.

Exactly as in Section 3.1, the corresponding eigenvectors $e(\Lambda_1(\omega))$ and $e(\Lambda_2(\omega))$ define the splitting of the tangent bundle of the sphere S^5 similar to (3.3.1):

$$TS^5 = \theta^1_R \oplus \eta^1_{\mathbb{C}}(e(\Lambda_1)) \oplus \eta^1_{\mathbb{C}}(e(\Lambda_2)),$$

where θ^1_R is the trivial one-dimensional real vector bundle tangent to the $U(1)$-orbits on S^5, as in (3.3.1), and one-dimensional complex vector bundles $\eta^1_{\mathbb{C}}(e(\Lambda_1))$ and $\eta^1_{\mathbb{C}}(e(\Lambda_2))$ correspond to the directions of the eigenvectors $e(\Lambda_1(\omega))$ and $e(\Lambda_2(\omega))$, respectively.

Hence, in the complex space $\mathbb{C}^3$, for any pair of convex bodies from the example (3.1.5) there is a two-dimensional complex plane $P^2_{\mathbb{C}} \subset \mathbb{C}^3$ such that the projections of these bodies V_1 and V_2 onto this plane are four-dimensional balls: $|z_1|^2+|z_2|^2 \leq \text{const}$. As in the real case, the transformation $\varphi \in SU(2)$ cannot be well defined here.

The next theorem is established by induction on the dimension n.

Theorem 3.3.2. *Let V_1 and V_2 be compact convex bodies in $\mathbb{C}^n$, $n \geq 3$, such that*

(1) *their projections* $V_1(P^2_{\mathbb{C}})$ *and* $V_2(P^2_{\mathbb{C}})$ *onto any two-dimensional complex plane* $P^2_{\mathbb{C}} \subset \mathbb{C}^n$ *are* $SU(2)$*-congruent and have no* $SU(2)$*-symmetries,*

(2) *for each of these bodies, its projections onto different complex lines are pairwise noncongruent with respect to the group* $U(1)$ *and have no* $U(1)$*-symmetries.*

Then the bodies V_1 *and* V_2 *are either parallel or centrally symmetric to each other in* $\mathbb{C}^n$.

It is worth recalling that in the proofs of Theorems 3.3.1 and 3.3.2 we did not make any calculations with the support of the width functions of the bodies V_1 and V_2, as it was done for the real case in Chapter 2. The only numerical characteristic which was considered in this section was the matrix M_0.

Note also that the conditions of $SU(2)$-congruence of projections of the bodies V_1 and V_2 onto **all** two-dimensional complex planes in $\mathbb{C}^n$ were essentially used in the proofs of these theorems. Excessive reduction of such projection data in these theorems is impossible, which is shown by the following purely algebraic example:

Let V be a compact convex body in a complex vector space $\mathbb{C}^{2n}$, where the standard quaternionic structure is introduced. It is well known that the groups $SU(2)$ and $Sp(1)$ are isomorphic. Given any non-identity element $g \in Sp(1)$, consider the body $g(V) \subset H^n = \mathbb{C}^{2n}$, which is obtained by the action of this transformation g on the points of the body V.

It is obvious that the projections of the bodies $g(V)$ and V onto any quaternionic line in H^n are transformed into each other by the action of this element $g \in Sp(1)$. If the body V is sufficiently asymmetric, then the bodies $g(V)$ and V are neither parallel nor centrally symmetric to each other.

In this example, the "quaternionic" projection data are described by the quaternionic projective space HP^{n-1}, which has dimension $4n-4$ while the complex Grassmann manifold $CG_{2,2n-2}$ of all two-dimensional complex planes in $\mathbb{C}^{2n}$ has dimension $8n-8$.

Analogous example disproves the attempts to "economize" on the real projection data in Theorems 2.1.1 and 2.1.2.

Let $V \subset \mathbb{R}^{2n} = \mathbb{C}^n$ be a compact convex body and let $g \in SO(2) = U(1)$ be any non-identity element. Then the bodies $g(V)$ and V have g-congruent projections onto any complex line, but in general these bodies are not necessarily parallel or centrally symmetric to each other. As above, in this example the complex projection data are described by the complex projective space CP^{n-1}, which has dimension two times lower than that of the real projection data, $RG_{2,2n-2}$.

The results obtained above can be generalized to the case of $(n-2)$-visible and $(n-2)$-convex compact bodies in $\mathbb{C}^n$, $n \geq 3$. In the next theorem the notion *convex hull* will be regarded in the classical sense as in the real vector space.

Theorem 3.3.3. *Let W_1 and W_2 be compact $(n-2)$-convex bodies in $\mathbb{C}^n$, $n \geq 3$, such that*

(1) their projections $W_1(P^2_{\mathbb{C}})$ and $W_2(P^2_{\mathbb{C}})$ onto any two-dimensional complex plane $P^2_{\mathbb{C}} \subset \mathbb{C}^n$ are $SU(2)$-congruent and the convex hulls of these projections have no $SU(2)$-symmetries,

(2) for each of these bodies, the convex hulls of its projections onto different complex lines are pairwise noncongruent with respect to the group $U(1)$ and have no symmetries with respect to this group.

Then the bodies W_1 and W_2 are either parallel or centrally symmetric to each other in $\mathbb{C}^n$.

The proof of this theorem is based on the fact that the convex hulls of these bodies W_1 and W_2 satisfy the assumptions of Theorem 3.3.1.

Theorem 3.3.4. *Let $W_1, W_2 \subset \mathbb{C}^n$, $n \geq 3$, be compact $(n-2)$-visible bodies such that*

(1) their projections $W_1(P^2_{\mathbb{C}})$ and $W_2(P^2_{\mathbb{C}})$ onto any two-dimensional complex plane $P^2_{\mathbb{C}} \subset \mathbb{C}^n$ are $SU(2)$-congruent and have no $SU(2)$-symmetries,

(2) for each of these bodies, its projections onto different complex lines are pairwise noncongruent with respect to the group $U(1)$ and have no symmetries with respect to this group.

Then the bodies W_1 and W_2 are either parallel or centrally symmetric to each other in $\mathbb{C}^n$.

Proof. The proof of this theorem is carried out by induction on the dimension n and is based on the fact that the projection of $(n-2)$-visible compact body on any complex hyperplane in $\mathbb{C}^n$ is an $(n-3)$-visible body in this hyperplane. Thus, we reduce this theorem to the case $n = 3$. Since the projections of the bodies W_1 and W_2 onto any two-dimensional complex plane in $\mathbb{C}^n$ have no $SU(2)$-symmetries, we can define a continuous mapping $\varphi : S^5 \longrightarrow SU(2)$ exactly in the same way as in Theorem 3.3.1 for the case of convex bodies. The rest of the proof of our theorem literally repeats that of Theorem 3.3.1. □

Note that, in contrast with the real analogue of this theorem, we do not require here the simple connectedness of the objects under consideration. As was mentioned above, the proofs of our theorems in the complex spaces follow from the considerations of the mapping φ only.

Exactly as in Section 2.3, Theorem 3.3.3 about $(n-2)$-convex bodies and Theorem 3.3.4 about $(n-2)$-visible bodies in $\mathbb{C}^n$ do not follow from each other because the conditions (1) and (2) in Theorem 2.3.1 are stronger than those of Theorem 2.3.2, and on the other hand, not any $(n-2)$-convex body in $\mathbb{C}^n$ is $(n-2)$-visible.

The examples constructed in Petty and McKinney (1987), Gardner and Volčič (1994) (see Section 3.1) for the case of real Euclidean spaces demonstrate that in these theorems it is apparently impossible to completely avoid the conditions of the absence of symmetries of the projections.

Theorems 3.3.1, 3.3.2 and their nonconvex analogues can be generalized to the cases of $U(2)$ and other unitary transformations of projections of the bodies in $\mathbb{C}^n$, $n \geq 3$.

Theorem 3.3.5. *Let V_1 and V_2 be compact convex bodies in $\mathbb{C}^n$, $n \geq 3$, such that*

(1) their projections $V_1(P^2_{\mathbb{C}})$ and $V_2(P^2_{\mathbb{C}})$ onto any two-dimensional complex plane $P^2_{\mathbb{C}} \subset \mathbb{C}^n$ are $U(2)$-congruent and have no $U(2)$-symmetries,

(2) for each of these bodies, its projections onto different complex lines are pairwise noncongruent with respect to the group $U(1)$ and have no $U(1)$-symmetries.

Then the bodies V_1 and V_2 are either parallel in $\mathbb{C}^n$ or directly homothetic, and the modulus of their homothety coefficient equals one.

Actually, this means that the bodies V_1 and V_2 are $U(1)$-congruent in $\mathbb{C}^n$.

Proof. Similarly to the case of $SO(2)$ and $SU(2)$-congruent projections, we shall start from the consideration of 3-dimensional ambient space $\mathbb{C}^3$.

As in the proof of Theorem 3.3.1, for any unit vector $\omega_0 \in S^5 \subset \mathbb{C}^3$ the $U(2)$-transformation $\varphi(\omega_0)$ of the projection $V_2(\omega_0)$ into $V_1(\omega_0)$ in the plane $P(\omega_0)$ is described by the matrix

$$M(\omega_0) = \begin{pmatrix} \exp(\mathrm{i}\lambda_1(\omega_0)) & 0 \\ 0 & \exp(\mathrm{i}\lambda_2(\omega_0)) \end{pmatrix}, \tag{3.3.2}$$

in some orthonormal basis $\{e_1(\omega_0), e_2(\omega_0)\}$ of this plane. Given any unit vector $\omega_1 \in P(e_2(\omega_0))$, consider the transformation $\varphi(\omega_1)$ of the projection $V_2(\omega_1)$ into $V_1(\omega_1)$. Let $e_1'(\omega_0)$ be a unit vector orthogonal to ω_1 and $e_2(\omega_0)$.

Lemma 3.3.2. *The transformation $\varphi(\omega_1)$ of the plane $P(\omega_1)$ in the orthonormal basis $\{e_1'(\omega_0), e_2(\omega_0)\}$ is described by the diagonal matrix*

$$M(\omega_1) = \begin{pmatrix} \exp(\mathrm{i}\lambda_1(\omega_1)) & 0 \\ 0 & \exp(\mathrm{i}\lambda_2(\omega_0)) \end{pmatrix}.$$

Proof. The proof of this lemma repeats that of Lemma 3.3.1. Note that, in contrast with the $SU(2)$-case, here the first eigenvalues of the matrices $M(\omega_0)$ and $M(\omega_1)$ can be different, while their second eigenvalues coincide. □

Now, we continue the proof of Theorem 3.3.5. Consider the particular case $\omega_1 = e_1(\omega_0)$ of the previous lemma. Suppose that the diagonal elements of the matrix $M(e_1(\omega_0))$ are not equal: $\exp(\mathrm{i}\lambda_1(e_1(\omega_0))) \neq \exp(\mathrm{i}\lambda_2(e_1(\omega_0)))$. It follows from Lemma 3.3.2 that for any unit vector $\omega_2 \in P(e_1(\omega_0))$ which is not parallel to ω_0 and to $e_2(\omega_0)$ the transformations $\varphi(\omega_2)$ and $\varphi(e_2(\omega_2))$ of the planes $P(\omega_2)$ and $P(e_2(\omega_2))$ are described by the diagonal matrices of the form (3.3.2) in the orthonormal bases $\{e_1(\omega_0), e_2(\omega_2)\}$ and $\{e_1(\omega_0), \omega_2\}$, respectively. Moreover, for any coordinate plane of the bases $B_0 = \{\omega_0, e_1(\omega_0), e_2(\omega_0)\}$ and $B_2 = \{\omega_2, e_1(\omega_0), e_2(\omega_2)\}$ in $\mathbb{C}^3$, the corresponding matrix of the transformations $\varphi(\omega)$ is diagonal in one of these bases.

On the other hand, the plane $P(e_1(\omega_0))$ spanned on the vectors ω_0 and $e_2(\omega_0)$ (or ω_2 and $e_2(\omega_2)$) is the coordinate plane for each of these bases B_1 and B_2. Clearly, the matrix $M(e_1(\omega_0))$ is diagonal in these two different coordinate systems; hence, it should be a scalar matrix $M(e_1(\omega_0)) = \exp(\mathrm{i}\lambda(\omega_0)) \cdot E$.

In the same way, $M(e_2(\omega_0))$ should be a scalar matrix as well. Since the vector ω_0 has been chosen arbitrarily, one can verify that for any two-dimensional complex plane $P(\omega) \subset \mathbb{C}^3$ the corresponding transformation

$\varphi(\omega) : V_2(\omega) \longrightarrow V_1(\omega)$ is described by a scalar matrix, i. e., it is a homothety with complex coefficient $\exp(\mathrm{i}\lambda(\omega))$. It follows from condition (2) of our theorem and Lemma 1.2.4 that the bodies V_1 and V_2 are homothetic in $\mathbb{C}^3$ with the same homothety coefficient.

For higher-dimensional complex Euclidean spaces $\mathbb{C}^n$ our theorem can be proved by induction on the dimension n as above. □

The next theorem follows from Theorem 3.3.3 and the previous one.

Theorem 3.3.6. *Let W_1 and W_2 be compact $(n-2)$-convex bodies in $\mathbb{C}^n$, $n \geq 3$, such that*

(1) their projections $W_1(P^2_{\mathbb{C}})$ and $W_2(P^2_{\mathbb{C}})$ onto any two-dimensional complex plane $P^2_{\mathbb{C}} \subset \mathbb{C}^n$ are $U(2)$-congruent and the convex hulls of these projections have no $U(2)$-symmetries,

(2) for each of these bodies, the convex hulls of its projections onto different complex lines are pairwise noncongruent with respect to the group $U(1)$ and have no symmetries with respect to this group.

Then the bodies W_1 and W_2 are either parallel or directly homothetic in $\mathbb{C}^n$, and the modulus of their homothety coefficient equals one.

If the projections of two bodies $W_1, W_2 \subset \mathbb{C}^n$ onto any two-dimensional plane $P^2_{\mathbb{C}} \subset \mathbb{C}^n$ are $U(2)$-congruent and have no $U(2)$-symmetries, then the unitary transformation of this plane $\varphi(P^2_{\mathbb{C}}) : W_2(P^2_{\mathbb{C}}) \longrightarrow W_1(P^2_{\mathbb{C}})$ is well defined, as above. Hence, a similar statement holds for $(n-2)$-visible bodies in $\mathbb{C}^n$ as well.

In contrast with the real case, any unitary $k \times k$ matrix has diagonal form in some orthonormal basis of the complex space $\mathbb{C}^k$. Therefore, our previous results can be extended to the case of compact convex bodies in $\mathbb{C}^n$ which have $U(k)$-congruent projections onto any k-dimensional complex plane, $k > 2$.

Theorem 3.3.7. *Let V_1 and V_2 be compact convex bodies in $\mathbb{C}^n$, $n \geq 3$, such that*

(1) their projections $V_1(P^2_{\mathbb{C}})$ and $V_2(P^2_{\mathbb{C}})$ onto any k-dimensional complex plane $P^k_{\mathbb{C}} \subset \mathbb{C}^n$, $n > k \geq 2$, are $U(k)$-congruent and have no $U(k)$-symmetries,

(2) for each of these bodies, its projections onto different $(k-1)$-dimensional complex planes are pairwise noncongruent and have no $U(1)$-symmetries.

Then the bodies V_1 and V_2 are either parallel in $\mathbb{C}^n$ or directly homothetic, and the modulus of their homothety coefficient equals one.

Again we begin with the case $n = k + 1$. For any unit vector $\omega_0 \in S^{2n-1}$, the transformation $\varphi(\omega_0) \in U(n-1)$ of the projection $V_2(\omega_0)$ into $V_1(\omega_0)$ in the complex hyperplane $P^k_{\mathbb{C}}(\omega_0)$ is represented by a diagonal matrix $M(\omega_0)$ with eigenvalues $\exp(\mathrm{i}\lambda_1(\omega_0)), \ldots, \exp(\mathrm{i}\lambda_k(\omega_0))$ in some orthonormal basis $B_0 = \{e_1(\omega_0), \ldots, e_k(\omega_0)\}$ of this hyperplane. As above, consider any orthonormal basis $\{\omega_1, e_1'(\omega_1)\}$ in the coordinate plane $O, \omega_0, e_1(\omega_0)$ of B_0 and the corresponding unitary transformation $\varphi(\omega_1) : V_2(\omega_1) \longrightarrow V_1(\omega_1)$.

Lemma 3.3.3. *Under the hypotheses of Theorem 3.3.7, the transformation $\varphi(\omega_1)$ of the complex hyperplane $P(\omega_1)$ is described by a diagonal matrix with elements $\exp(\mathrm{i}\mu(\omega_1))$, $\exp(\mathrm{i}\lambda_2(\omega_0)), \ldots,$ $\exp(\mathrm{i}\lambda_k(\omega_0))$ in the orthonormal basis $B_1 = \{e_1'(\omega_1), e_2(\omega_0), \ldots, e_k(\omega_0)\}$.*

Proof. The proof of this lemma reproduces that of Lemma 3.3.1.

If the unitary matrix $M(\omega_1)$ is not diagonal in this basis, then some of its lines contains nonzero nondiagonal elements. Without loss of generality we can assume that it is the first line of this matrix. Obviously, in this case the $(k-1)$-dimensional plane $P_1^{k-1} \subset P(\omega_1)$ spanned on the vectors $e_2(\omega_1), \ldots, e_k(\omega_0)$ is not parallel to the plane $\varphi(\omega_1)(P_1^{k-1})$.

As in the case $k = 2$, the projections of the bodies V_1 and V_2 onto the plane P_1^{k-1} are $U(k-1)$-congruent and their projections onto the hyperplane $P(\omega_1)$ are $U(k)$-congruent. Hence, the projections of the body V_1 onto different $(k-1)$-dimensional planes P_1^{k-1} and $\varphi(\omega_1)(P_1^{k-1})$ are $U(k-1)$-congruent:

$$V_1(P_1^{k-1}) \sim V_2(P_1^{k-1}) \sim V_1(\varphi(\omega_1)(P_1^{k-1})),$$

which contradicts condition (2) of our theorem. □

Proof of Theorem 3.3.7. Suppose that the eigenvalues of the diagonal matrix $M(\omega_0)$ do not coincide, say,

$$\exp(\mathrm{i}\lambda_1(\omega_0)) \neq \exp(\mathrm{i}\lambda_2(\omega_0)). \tag{3.3.3}$$

Consider any orthonormal basis $\{\omega_1, e_1'(\omega_1)\}$ in the coordinate plane O, ω_0, $e_1(\omega_0)$ and a similar basis $\{\omega_2, e_1'(\omega_2)\}$ in the coordinate plane O, ω_0, $e_0(\omega_0)$. We shall assume that the vectors ω_1 and ω_2 are not parallel to the vectors that constitute the basis B_0. It follows from the previous lemma that the transformations $\varphi(\omega_1)$ and $\varphi(\omega_2)$ are described by diagonal matrices in the bases B_1 and $B_2 = \{e_1(\omega_0), e_2'(\omega_2), e_3(\omega_0), \dots, e_k(\omega_0)\}$, respectively.

If we reproduce this construction for $\omega_0' = e_1(\omega_0)$ (or for $\omega_0' = e_2(\omega_0)$), then the previous lemma implies that for any orthonormal basis $\{\omega_3, e_2'(\omega_3)\}$ in the coordinate plane O, $e_1(\omega_0)$, $e_2(\omega_0)$ the matrix $M(\omega_0)$ should be diagonal in the basis B_0 and in the basis $B_3 = \{\omega_3, e_2'(\omega_0), e_3(\omega_2), \dots, e_k(\omega_0)\}$ simultaneously. Since the vector ω_3 can be chosen arbitrarily in this coordinate plane, the eigenvalues of the matrix $M(\omega_0)$ that correspond to this plane should be equal. Exactly as in the case $k = 2$, this contradicts the assumption (3.3.3).

For the higher-dimensional spaces $\mathbb{C}^n$, $n > k + 1$, our theorem can be proved by induction on n. □

In a similar way as above, this theorem can be formulated for the $(n-k)$-visible and $(n-k)$-convex bodies $W_1, W_2 \subset \mathbb{C}^n$ whose projections onto any k-dimensional plane in $\mathbb{C}^n$, $n \geq 3$, $n > k \geq 2$, are $U(k)$-congruent and the convex hulls of these projections (or these projections themselves) do not have $U(k)$-symmetries (cf. Theorem 3.3.6).

Chapter 4.

Apparent contours and other tomography-type projection data

4.1. RECONSTRUCTION OF SURFACES FROM THE SHAPES OF THEIR APPARENT CONTOURS AND THE STATIONARY PHASE OBSERVATIONS

The main results of this section concern the classical problem that we have studied in the previous chapters: if two surfaces in the Euclidean space have congruent projections onto any plane, how different can they be?

Here we consider the apparent contours of the smooth hypersurfaces as the projection data and formulate some sufficient conditions of coincidence of the shapes of two hypersurfaces if the shapes of their apparent contours on any two-dimensional plane coincide. We also obtain new results on reconstruction of smooth surfaces from the observations of the wave fronts generated by these surfaces. Most of the results presented here were obtained in the joint paper Golubyatnikov *et al.* (1999a).

(a) As above, we denote by $P(\omega)$ the oriented hyperplane with unit normal vector ω in the Euclidean space $\mathbb{R}^n$, $n \geq 2$. Let $M^{n-1} \subset \mathbb{R}^n$ be a compact smooth closed hypersurface.

Following Haefliger (1960) and Pointet (1997), the set of the points $y \in P(\omega)$ such that the straight line containing y and orthogonal to $P(\omega)$ is tangent to M^{n-1} at some point $m(y)$ will be called *the apparent contour* of

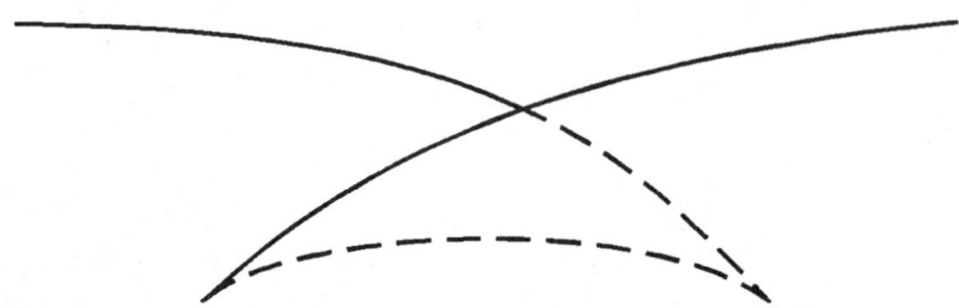

Figure 4.1: An apparent contour of Saint-Exupérie's surface

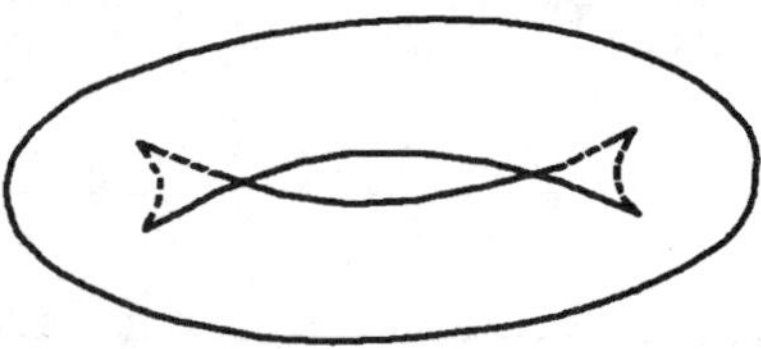

Figure 4.2: An apparent contour of the standard torus of revolution. See Haefliger (1960) and Pignoni (1991) for more queer examples

the surface M^{n-1} in the direction ω and will be denoted by $C(M, \omega)$. Beside these points $m(y)$, each of these lines can intersect the hypersurface M^{n-1} transversally finitely many times (see Figures 4.1 and 4.2).

It is very easy to see that for a convex smooth surface $M^{n-1} \subset \mathbb{R}^n$ its apparent contour in any hyperplane $P(\omega)$ is just the boundary of the orthogonal projection of M^{n-1} onto this plane $P(\omega)$.

Pointet has shown that if the apparent contours $C(M_1, \omega)$ and $C(M_2, \omega)$ of smooth hypersurfaces $M_1, M_2 \subset \mathbb{R}^n$ coincide for a sufficiently large set W of directions $\omega \in S^{n-1}$, then these hypersurfaces coincide themselves. The condition on such a set W was formulated in Pointet (1997) as follows:

For any hyperplane $P \in \mathbb{R}^n$ containing the zero point, its intersection with $W \subset S^{n-1}$ is nonempty and for all quadratic forms Q over P the equality $Q(\omega) = 0$ for all $\omega \in P \cap W$ implies that Q is degenerate.

Pointet calls these sets n-omnidirectional.

Such apparent contours projection data have a natural physical interpretation: if a thin-walled transparent membrane M is examined by the laser beams, X-rays or other high-frequency radiation, the signals spreading along the rays tangent to the inner surface of the membrane lose much more energy

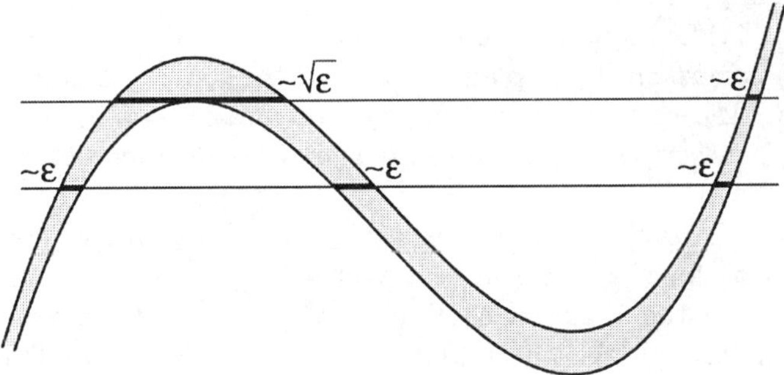

Figure 4.3: Transversal and tangent intersections of a membrane with straight lines

than those which have only transversal intersections with this membrane, as in Figure 4.3. Analogous well-known pictures appear naturally in various domains of pure and applied mathematics (see, for example, Spivak, 1990). This phenomenon can be easily reproduced with the help of an overhead and a sheet of transparent film.

Another very useful case of the apparent contours observations is connected with the phase shift of the signals spreading along the rays tangent to the caustics. This effect is well known in the theory of seismic waves propagation and is explained by the stationary phase method.

In the particular case $n = 2$, using the dual numbers formalism (Pekmen, 1995), one can construct some useful numerical characteristics of the apparent contours, such as

$$\oint_{C(M^2,\omega)} \langle \nu, \omega, \,\mathrm{d}y\rangle = I(\nu, \omega, M^2),$$

where ν is the unit normal to M^2 at the point $m(y)$, $y \in C(M^2, \omega)$, $\mathrm{d}y$ is the length differential of this contour, and $\langle\cdot\,,\cdot\,,\cdot\rangle$ denotes the scalar triple product of the vectors $\nu, \omega, \mathrm{d}y$. This integral $I(\nu, \omega, M^2)$ is equal to the alternating sum of the lengths of the arcs of the contour $C(M^2, \omega)$ between its singular points and is directly connected to the Maslov index construction.

Using the results of Pointet and the methods developed in Chapter 2, we obtain the basic result of this section:

Theorem 4.1.1. *Let M_1 and M_2 be smooth closed compact surfaces in $\mathbb{R}^3$ such that for any $\omega \in S^2$ the apparent contours $C(M_1, \omega)$ and $C(M_2, \omega)$ are $SO(2)$-congruent in the plane $P(\omega)$, and the convex hulls* $\operatorname{conv} C(M_1, \omega)$ *and* $\operatorname{conv} C(M_2, \omega)$ *of these contours have no rotation symmetries. Then M_1 and M_2 are either parallel or centrally symmetric to each other.*

Proof. To prove the theorem, we define a map $\varphi : S^2 \longrightarrow S^1$ as in Section 2.1 as follows: given a unit vector $\omega \in S^2$, let $\varphi(\omega) \in S^1$ be the angle such that the apparent contour $C(M_2, \omega)$ is obtained from $C(M_1, \omega)$ by rotation through the angle $\varphi(\omega)$. Note that the convex hulls of these contours are congruent with respect to the same rotations.

As in Section 2.1, the asymmetry of the convex hulls of these contours implies that this map is well defined and continuous.

Applying Theorem 2.1.1 to the convex hulls $\operatorname{conv} M_1$ and $\operatorname{conv} M_2$ of the surfaces M_1 and M_2, we see that these convex hulls are either parallel or centrally symmetric to each other in $\mathbb{R}^3$. The transformation that carries $\operatorname{conv} M_2$ onto $\operatorname{conv} M_1$ carries the surface M_2 into some surface M_2' such that

(1) $\operatorname{conv} M_2' = \operatorname{conv} M_1$;

(2) for any $\omega \in S^2$ the apparent contours $C(M_2', \omega)$ and $C(M_1, \omega)$ are $SO(2)$-congruent.

Assume that for some $\omega_0 \in S^2$ we have $C(M_2', \omega) \neq C(M_1, \omega)$, i. e., $C(M_2', \omega)$ is transformed into $C(M_1, \omega)$ by a non-identical isometry g. It follows from condition (1) that for any $\omega \in S^2$ $\operatorname{conv} C(M_2', \omega) = \operatorname{conv} C(M_1, \omega)$. Hence, these convex hulls are transformed into each other by two different mappings: by the identity map and by g, which is impossible, since these convex hulls have no $SO(2)$-symmetries.

Thus, the apparent contours of the surfaces M_1 and M_2' coincide in all directions and the results of Pointet (1997) imply the coincidence of these surfaces. $\square$

Theorem 4.1.2. *Let M_1 and M_2 be smooth compact closed surfaces in $\mathbb{R}^3$. If for all $\omega \in S^2$ their apparent contours $C(M_1, \omega)$ and $C(M_2, \omega)$ are $SO(2)$-similar and their convex hulls* $\operatorname{conv} C(M_1, \omega)$ *and* $\operatorname{conv} C(M_2, \omega)$ *have no $SO(2)$-symmetries (as in Section 3.1, the ratio of the similitude is not supposed to be constant, independent of the plane $P(\omega)$), then these surfaces M_1 and M_2 in R^3 are either parallel or directly homothetic.*

Proof. As in Section 3.1, the proof of this theorem is carried out in two steps:

(1) we prove that the convex hulls $\operatorname{conv} C(M_1, \omega)$ and $\operatorname{conv} C(M_2, \omega)$ are equivalent either with respect to a homothety H or with respect to a parallel translation T;

(2) since the convex hulls of the projections of the apparent contours of the surfaces M_1, M_2 have no $SO(2)$-symmetries, then after one of these transformations H or T the apparent contours $C(M_1, \omega)$ and $C(M_2, \omega)$ coincide for all $\omega \in S^2$. Now, using the theorem of Pointet we establish the coincidence of the surface M_2 and the surface M_1', obtained from M_1 by one of the transformations H or T.

□

Theorems 4.1.1 and 4.1.2 have analogues in the higher-dimensional spaces.

These considerations do not seem to be too artificial from the practical viewpoint, because the projections images sometimes have much more complicated structure than a curve on the display of a computer. Many physical phenomena connected with the wave fronts transformations (caustics, the focus points, etc.) usually are studied as the singularities of projections of hypersurfaces in the 6-dimensional phase space onto the configuration manifold $\mathbb{R}^3$ (see Arnol'd *et al.*, 1985; Arnol'd, 1978).

In order to describe the projections of smooth hypersurfaces $M^{n-1} \subset \mathbb{R}^n$ onto $(n-k)$-dimensional planes for $k \geq 1$, we recall some useful definitions.

Let $G_{n,k}$ be the Grassmann manifold of all k-dimensional subspaces in $\mathbb{R}^n$. For any $x \in G_{n,k}$ we denote by $x^\perp \in G_{n,n-k}$ its orthogonal complement.

Let $G : M^{n-1} \longrightarrow S^{n-1}$ be the Gauss map which associates any point of the surface with the unit normal vector at this point. Consider the orthogonal projection $p_x : M^{n-1} \longrightarrow x^\perp$ along the k-dimensional plane x, and let $\Sigma(p_x) = G^{-1}(x^\perp \cap S^{n-1})$ be the set of critical points of this projection. The set $C(M, x) = p_x(\Sigma(p_x))$ is called *the apparent contour of the hypersurface M^{n-1} in the direction x.*

It is easy to verify that $C(M, x)$ consists of the points $y \in x^\perp$ such that the k-dimensional plane containing y and parallel to x is tangent to M^{n-1} at some point.

The following definition and theorem belong to Pointet (1997):

Definition. Given $W \subset G_{n,k}$, we say that W is n^k-omnidirectional if for all hyperplanes π there exists $w \in W$ with $w \subset \pi$, and if for any quadratic form Q over π, $Q|_w$ degenerates for all $w \in W$ with $w \subset \pi$, then Q is degenerate.

Theorem. *If the apparent contours $C(M_1, x)$, $C(M_2, x)$ of smooth hypersurfaces $M_1, M_2 \subset \mathbb{R}^n$ coincide for an n^k-omnidirectional set $W \subset G_{n,k}$ of k-dimensional planes, then these hypersurfaces coincide themselves.*

First, we consider the apparent contours of the surfaces in two-dimensional planes.

Theorem 4.1.3. *Let M_1 and M_2 be smooth closed compact hypersurfaces in $\mathbb{R}^n$, $n \geq 2$, such that for any $(n-2)$-dimensional subspace $x \in G_{n,2}$ the apparent contours $C(M_1, x^\perp)$, $C(M_2, x^\perp)$ are $SO(2)$-congruent in $x^\perp$, and the convex hulls $\operatorname{conv} C(M_1, x^\perp)$ and $\operatorname{conv} C(M_2, x^\perp)$ of these contours have no $SO(2)$-symmetries. Then the surfaces M_1 and M_2 are either parallel or centrally symmetric to each other.*

Theorem 4.1.4. *Let M_1 and M_2 be smooth closed compact hypersurfaces in $\mathbb{R}^n$, $n \geq 2$, such that for any $(n-2)$-dimensional subspace $x \in G_{n,2}$ the apparent contours $C(M_1, x^\perp)$ and $C(M_2, x^\perp)$ are $SO(2)$-similar and the convex hulls $\operatorname{conv} C(M_1, x^\perp)$ and $\operatorname{conv} C(M_2, x^\perp)$ of these contours have no $SO(2)$-symmetries. Then the surfaces M_1 and M_2 are either parallel or directly homothetic.*

Proof. Both of these theorems, as Theorem 4.1.2, are proved in two steps:

(1) we prove that for all $x \in G_{n,2}$ the convex hulls $\operatorname{conv} C(M_1, x^\perp)$ and $\operatorname{conv} C(M_2, x^\perp)$ are equivalent with respect to either a homothety H or a parallel translation T or a central symmetry S;

(2) the condition of asymmetry of these convex hulls imply that they are congruent with respect to one of these transformations H, S or T, and the assertions of our theorems follow from Pointet (1997), Theorem 13.

□

Similar considerations can be reproduced for the apparent contours $C(M, x^{\perp})$, $x \in G_{n,3}$ in three-dimensional planes in $\mathbb{R}^n$, using the results and methods developed in Section 3.2.

Theorem 4.1.5. *Let M_1 and M_2 be smooth closed compact hypersurfaces in $\mathbb{R}^n$, $n \geq 4$, such that*

(1) the apparent contours $C(M_1, x^{\perp})$ and $C(M_2, x^{\perp})$ in every three-dimensional subspace $x^{\perp}$ are $SO(3)$-congruent with respect to some orientation-preserving isometry $\mathbf{s}(x^{\perp})$ of the plane $x^{\perp}$;

(2) the convex hulls $\operatorname{conv} C(M_1, x^{\perp})$ and $\operatorname{conv} C(M_2, x^{\perp})$ of these contours have no $SO(3)$-symmetries, and the width functions of $\operatorname{conv} M_1$, $\operatorname{conv} M_2$ have finitely many maxima.

Then the surfaces M_1 and M_2 are parallel in $\mathbb{R}^n$.

A similar theorem holds for the isometry $\mathbf{s}(x^{\perp})$ which does not preserve the orientation of the planes $x^{\perp}$ (cf. Golubyatnikov, 1995a).

Theorem 4.1.6. *Let M_1 and M_2 be smooth, closed and compact hypersurfaces in $\mathbb{R}^n$, $n \geq 4$, such that*

(1) the apparent contours $C(M_1, x^{\perp})$ and $C(M_2, x^{\perp})$ in every three-dimensional subspace $x^{\perp}$ are $SO(3)$-similar;

(2) the convex hulls $\operatorname{conv} C(M_1, x^{\perp})$ and $\operatorname{conv} C(M_2, x^{\perp})$ of these contours have no $SO(3)$-symmetries and the width functions of $\operatorname{conv} M_1$ and $\operatorname{conv} M_2$ have finitely many maxima.

Then M_1 and M_2 are either parallel in $\mathbb{R}^n$ or directly homothetic with positive coefficient.

Proof. This theorem is reduced to the previous one by means of the homothety of M_1 with coefficient equal to the ratio of the diameters of the hypersurfaces M_1 and M_2. □

Analogous statement holds for the similarities that do not preserve the orientation of $x^{\perp}$; in this case the initial hypersurfaces are equivalent with respect to some homothety with negative coefficient.

(b) Reconstruction of the surfaces from the exponential maps of their normal bundles.

The apparent contours projection data are connected with the natural map

$$G : STM^{n-1} \longrightarrow TS^{n-1}$$

of the spherical subbundle of the tangent bundle of the hypersurface M^{n-1} to the tangent bundle of the unit sphere, which plays the role of the oriented Grassmann manifold here. Namely, given $x \in M^{n-1}$ and a unit vector ω tangent to M^{n-1} at the point x, one defines $G(x, \omega)$ as the intersection of the line $X = x + t\omega$ with the plane tangent to the unit sphere $S^{n-1} \subset \mathbb{R}^n$ at the point ω; in other words, this is the foot of the corresponding perpendicular. In contrast with these projections in the directions of the tangent vectors, we consider here the dual case, which is associated with the map

$$G^{\perp} : SNM \longrightarrow S^{n-1}$$

of the spherical subbundle of the normal bundle of the manifold M immersed in $\mathbb{R}^n$. From the physical viewpoint, it is natural to generalize this situation to the non-Euclidean spaces. So, the end of this section is devoted to the reconstruction of a manifold M immersed into a Riemannian manifold with boundary from the information about the wave fronts generated by this manifold M (or exponential map of its normal bundle), measured on this boundary. The projection data of this type appear in the kinematic problems of seismology or seismic tomography (see Gol'din, 1997) and in the modelling of the earthquakes sources.

A Riemannian metric g on a compact manifold B with boundary ∂B is called *simple* if every pair of points $p, q \in B$ can be joined by the unique geodesic line $\gamma_{p,q}$ of this metric whose all points with the possible exception of its endpoints belong to the interior of B, and such $\gamma_{p,q}$ depends smoothly on p and q. We shall suppose that such a simple metric g is defined in the ball $B^n \subset \mathbb{R}^n$. The Riemannian metrics of this type are often considered in the inverse kinematic and dynamic problems of seismology (Anikonov, 1995; Gol'din, 1997), in tomography (Sharafutdinov, 1992) and in other wave fronts investigations (Arnol'd *et al.*, 1985).

As it was shown by purely homotopical methods in Golubyatnikov (1978), the simplicity of the Riemannian metric g can be verified using the boundary observations, i. e., if the condition of the uniqueness of the geodesic line $\gamma_{p,q}$ holds for every pair $p, q \in \partial B$ and this line depends smoothly on its endpoints, then the metric g is simple.

The Riemannian metric g on the manifold B^n induces the canonical isomorphism $g^* : TB^n \longrightarrow T^*B^n$ of the tangent and cotangent bundles of B^n and all its submanifolds.

Consider a smooth oriented manifold M^{n-1} immersed into the interior of the ball B^n endowed by a simple Riemannian metric. For any point $x \in M^{n-1}$, denote by $v(x)$ the unit vector of the exterior normal to M^{n-1} at the point x. Let $\gamma(x)$ be the geodesic line starting from this point in the direction $v(x)$ and let $d(x)$ be the distance between x and the boundary ∂B^n. It is easy to see that the positive function $d : M^{n-1} \longrightarrow \mathbb{R}^1$ is continuous.

Any geodesic line of a simple metric in B^n arrives to its boundary ∂B^n in both of its directions (see, for example, Sharafutdinov, 1992). Denote by $y(x) = \exp_x(d(x) \cdot v(x)) \in \partial B^n$ the intersection of the line $\gamma(x)$ and $\partial B^n = S^{n-1}$; here $\exp_x(\cdot)$ is the exponential map of the tangent space T_xB^n to B^n. Let $\mu(x) \in T_{y(x)}$ be the unit tangent vector to $\gamma(x)$ at the point $y(x)$. Consider the covector $\varkappa^*(x) = g^*(\mu(x)) \in T^*_{y(x)}S^{n-1}$ defined by $\varkappa^*(x)(w) = \langle w, \mu(x)\rangle$ for all $w \in T_{y(x)}S^{n-1}$; here $\langle \cdot, \cdot \rangle$ denotes the scalar product generated by the metric g. Such a covector plays the role of the gradient of the length $l(x)$ of the geodesic segment of $\gamma(x)$ between x and $y(x)$.

We define the map $Y : M^{n-1} \longrightarrow T^*S^{n-1}$ by the formula $Y(x) = (y(x), \varkappa^*(x))$.

Lemma 4.1.1. *The image $Y(M^{n-1})$ is a Lagrangian manifold in T^*S^{n-1}.*

The proof follows from the definition of the optical length of the geodesic lines as the generating function of a germ of a Lagrangian manifold, see Arnol'd *et al.* (1985).

Note that this image $Y(M^{n-1})$ can be interpreted as the trace of the wave front generated by $M^{n-1} \subset B^n$ and registered on the boundary ∂B^n.

Theorem 4.1.7. *Let M^{n-1} be a smooth oriented compact closed connected manifold immersed into the interior of the ball B^n. Assume that the image $Y(M^{n-1})$ has only transversal self-intersections in T^*S^{n-1}. Then this image and the location of the point $x_0 \in M^{n-1}$ of the minimum of the function d determine this hypersurface M^{n-1} uniquely.*

Proof. To prove this theorem, note that in some neighborhood of the point x_0 the hypersurface M^{n-1} is uniquely determined because the gradient of a function determines this function up to a constant summand.

The uniqueness of reconstruction of M^{n-1} "in the large" follows from its connectedness and compactness. □

This theorem can be extended to the cases of manifolds of higher codimensions. Consider a smooth, oriented, compact, closed and connected manifold M^k immersed into the interior of B^n as above, $1 \leq k < n$. Let NM^k be the normal bundle of M^k in $\mathbb{R}^n$, and let SNM^k be its spherical subbundle. Denote by SN_xM^k the $(n-1-k)$-dimensional unit sphere in N_xM^k which is the orthogonal complement of the tangent space T_xM^k of the manifold M^k at the point x.

Given a unit vector $\alpha \in SN_xM^k$, consider the geodesic line $\gamma(x, \alpha)$ starting from the point $x \in M^k$ in the direction $\alpha \perp T_xM^k$. Let

$$y(x, \alpha) = \exp_x(l(x, \alpha) \cdot \alpha)$$

be the intersection of this geodesic line with the boundary ∂B^n, where $l(x, \alpha)$ is the length of its arc between the points x and $y(x, \alpha)$. We define the maps

$$Y : SNM^k \longrightarrow T^*S^{n-1}, \quad Z : SNM^k \longrightarrow \partial B^n \times \mathbb{R}^1$$

by the formulas

$$Y(x, \alpha) = (y(x, \alpha); \varkappa^*(x, \alpha)), \quad Z(x, \alpha) = (y(x, \alpha); l(x, \alpha)).$$

Here the covector $\varkappa^*(x, \alpha) = g^*(\mu(x, \alpha)) \in T^*_{y(x,\alpha)}S^{n-1}$ is defined as above by the formula $\varkappa^*(x, \alpha)(w) = \langle w, \mu(x, \alpha) \rangle$ for all $w \in T_{y(x,\alpha)}S^{n-1}$, where $\mu(x, \alpha)$ is the unit tangent vector of the line $\gamma(x, \alpha)$ at the point $y(x, \alpha)$.

Theorem 4.1.8. *Let M^k be a smooth oriented compact closed connected manifold immersed into the interior of the ball B^n. Assume that the image $Y(SNM^k)$ has only transversal self-intersections in T^*S^{n-1}. Then this image and the location of the point $x_0 \in M^k$ of the minimum of the function d uniquely determine this manifold M^k.*

Theorem 4.1.9. *Let M^k be the same as above. Then the image $Z(SNM^k)$ uniquely determines this manifold in B^n.*

The proofs of these theorems are similar to that of Theorem 4.1.7, i. e., they are based on the theory of the wave fronts transformation (see Arnol'd *et al.*, 1985).

The results on the uniqueness of reconstruction of surfaces from the wave fronts observations were obtained in the situation of general position.

Simple examples show that in the case of nontransversal self-intersections of the traces of the wave fronts the assertions of Theorems 4.1.7 and 4.1.8 are not true.

4.2. INVERSION FORMULAE FOR INTEGRAL GEOMETRY PROBLEMS AND AN ALGORITHM OF COMPUTERIZED TOMOGRAPHY

A typical integral geometry problem consists in reconstruction of a finite or rapidly decreasing function defined in $\mathbb{R}^n$ from the values of its integrals along some collection of k-dimensional planes, $1 \le k < n$. The most important cases from the applications viewpoint, $k = n - 1$ and $k = 1$, correspond to the inversion of the Radon transform and to the tomography problems, respectively. Various inverse problems of this kind were investigated in Blagoveshchenskii (1986), Gel'fand and Graev (1968), Gel'fand *et al.* (1967, 1980), Helgason (1980) and Natterer (1986); see also the references cited there. In this section we obtain some inversion formulae for these integral geometry problems and describe numerical experiments and an algorithm of reconstruction of the shape of a body in $\mathbb{R}^n$ and its density from a small collection of its X-ray projections. This algorithm was constructed in cooperation with N. B. Ayupova, who made a series of corresponding numerical experiments (see Ayupova and Golubyatnikov, 1990).

Let $G_{n,k}$ be the Grassmann manifold of oriented k-dimensional subspaces in $\mathbb{R}^n$ and let $G_{n,k,x}$ be the Grassmann manifold of k-dimensional oriented planes in $\mathbb{R}^n$ that contain a point $x \in \mathbb{R}^n$. We denote by $\tilde{G}_{n,k}$ and $\tilde{G}_{n,k,x}$ the corresponding Grassmann manifolds of unoriented planes and we suppose in the sequel that all these manifolds are endowed with the standard Riemannian metric.

The manifold of all k-dimensional oriented planes in $\mathbb{R}^n$ is diffeomorphic to the space $E\gamma_{n-k}$ of canonical $(n-k)$-dimensional vector bundle $\pi : \gamma_{n-k} \longrightarrow G_{n,k}$; any k-dimensional plane $\Pi^k \subset \mathbb{R}^n$ corresponds to its normal vector which joins the origin in $\mathbb{R}^n$ and the intersection point $\Pi^k \cap P^{n-k}$, where P^{n-k} is the subspace in $\mathbb{R}^n$ orthogonal to Π^k. Similar diffeomorphisms can be constructed in the unoriented and in the complex variants as well.

Each smooth, rapidly decreasing function f defined on $\mathbb{R}^n$ generates a function g on the space $E\gamma_{n-k}$ and on its unoriented analogue as follows:

$$g(\Pi^k) = \int\limits_{\Pi^k} f(x)\,\mathrm{d}x = \int\limits_{\mathbb{R}^k} f(\alpha t + \beta)\,\mathrm{d}t. \tag{4.2.1}$$

Here the plane Π^k consists of points $x \in \mathbb{R}^n$ such that $x = \beta + \alpha_1 t^1 + \ldots + \alpha_k t^k$, where $\beta \in \mathbb{R}^n$, and $\alpha = \alpha_1, \ldots, \alpha_k$ is a k-frame in $\mathbb{R}^n$. Denote this integral transformation by $g = J_k(f)$.

The questions of solvability of the equation (4.2.1) were considered in Gel'fand *et al.* (1967, 1980), where for even k an explicit inversion formulae were obtained. Namely, for such dimensions k the closed differential forms $\varkappa_x g$ were constructed on the Grassmann manifolds $G_{n,k}$ so that the unknown function f can be represented in the terms of $g = J_k(f)$ as follows:

$$f(x)\,(-1)^{k/2}\,2\,.(2\pi)^k d(Z) = \int\limits_Z \varkappa_x g. \tag{4.2.2}$$

Here $d(Z)$ is the intersection index of the Euler cycle in the Grassmann manifold $G_{n,k,x}$ and the k-dimensional cycle Z which is the integration domain in the right-hand side of (4.2.2). For even k, this form $\varkappa_x g$ is antisymmetric with respect to the antipodal involution $\omega \longleftrightarrow -\omega$ and thus it cannot be transferred to the unoriented Grassmann manifold $\tilde{G}_{n,k,x}$. In terms of coordinates of the vectors $\alpha_1, \ldots, \alpha_k$ which constitute the frame α, this differential form is defined by

$$\varkappa_x g(\alpha, x) = (-1)^k \sum_{i_1,\ldots,i_k=1}^{n} \frac{\partial^k g(\alpha, x)}{\partial x^{i_1} \ldots x^{i_k}}\, \mathrm{d}\alpha_1^{i_1} \wedge \ldots \wedge \mathrm{d}\alpha_k^{i_k}. \tag{4.2.3}$$

It was noted in Gel'fand *et al.* (1980) that the corresponding differential operator $\varkappa_x$ can be represented as a composition of the first-order operators

$$\sum_{i=1}^{n} \frac{\partial}{\partial x^i}\, \mathrm{d}\alpha_j^i, \qquad j = 1, \ldots, n.$$

Therefore, the value of $\varkappa_x$ on any k-dimensional multivector in $G_{n,k,x}$ does not depend on the choice of a basis $\alpha_1, \ldots \alpha_k$ in the plane Π^k. Hence, if b^k is dual to $\varkappa_x g$ with respect to the standard Riemannian metric, then the $(n-k-1)k$-dimensional multivector B complementary to b^k splits into the exterior product of k copies of $(n-k-1)$-dimensional multivectors.

The main aim of this section is construction of a similar differential form for odd values of $k = \dim \Pi^k$. We start our considerations from the inversion of the Radon transform, i.e., from the case $k = n-1$, when the oriented Grassmann manifold $G_{n,1} = G_{n,n-1}$ is an $(n-1)$-dimensional sphere and its unoriented analogue is the projective space RP^{n-1}.

As was mentioned above, the manifold of all straight lines in $\mathbb{R}^n$ is diffeomorphic to the fiber space $E\gamma_{n-1}$, its dimension is equal to $(2n-2)$ and its stable tangent bundle splits:

$$\tau(E\gamma_{n-1}) \oplus p^*(\theta^1) \approx p^*(n\gamma_1 \oplus \gamma_{n-1}) \approx p^*[(n-1)\gamma_1 \oplus n\theta^1]. \tag{4.2.4}$$

Here $p : \gamma_{n-1} \longrightarrow RP^{n-1}$ is the canonical $(n-1)$-dimensional vector bundle over RP^{n-1} and θ^1 is the trivial line bundle. The stable tangent bundles of other Grassmann manifolds admit similar splittings (see Szczarba, 1964).

Following the general idea described in Gel'fand *et al.* (1967), we consider the Euler cycle C as the domain of integration in the inversion formula (4.2.2) for odd k as well. It can be represented as Schubert's cell $C(2, 3, \dots, k+1)$ whose closure has empty boundary both in the oriented and in the nonoriented case because it is composed of all k-dimensional planes of some $(k+1)$-dimensional linear subspace $E^{k+1} \subset \mathbb{R}^n$.

The normal bundles of the Euler cycles considered as closed submanifolds in the Grassmann manifolds $G_{n,k,x}$ and $\tilde{G}_{n,k,x}$ are split into a sum of k copies of $(n-k-1)$-dimensional vector bundles isomorphic to $\mathrm{Hom}_{\mathbb{R}^1}(\tau, \theta^1)$, where τ is the tangent bundle of the Euler cycle and the trivial bundle θ^1 is determined by any of the normals to E^{k+1} in the sequence of subspaces $E^k \subset E^{k+1} \subset \dots \subset \mathbb{R}^n$ which defines the standard decomposition of the Grassmann manifold into Schubert's cells. All these k summands correspond to the variations of vectors of the frame $(\alpha_1, \dots, \alpha_k)$ along the directions orthogonal to E^{k+1} and the variation of these vectors along this subspace E^{k+1} determine the tangent bundle to the Euler cycle C.

Similar splittings of the normal bundles in the Grassmann manifolds can be constructed on the $2k$-dimensional Schubert's cell $C(3, 4, \dots, k+2)$, on the $3k$-dimensional Schubert's cell $C(4, 5, \dots, k+3)$, etc. Here we study the simplest case when the dimension of the integration domain in the inversion formulae is minimal.

In the k-dimensional homology groups of these manifolds, this cycle C is the most interesting for the inversion of the integral transformation J_k because the intersection index $d(C)$ equals 1 and the integrals of $\varkappa_x g$ along other k-dimensional Schubert's cells $C(1, m_2, \dots, m_k)$ vanish. We recall that the dimension of these cells is calculated by the formula $(m_1-1)+(m_2-2)+(m_3-3)+\dots+(m_k-k)$.

As was shown in Gel'fand *et al.* (1980), for even $n = k+1$

$$f(x) = 2m_n \int\limits_{|\omega|=1} K(\omega, x)\, \mathrm{d}\omega, \tag{4.2.5}$$

where $m_n = (2\pi)^{-n}(-1)^{n/2-1}/2$ and $d\omega$ is the standard volume form on the unit sphere $S^{n-1} \subset \mathbb{R}^n$,

$$K(\omega, x) = V.P. \int_{-\infty}^{\infty} \frac{\partial^{n-1}\widehat{f}(\omega, s)}{\partial s^{n-1}}\bigg|_{s=q+<\omega,x>} q^{-1}\, dq.$$

Here $\widehat{f}$ is the Radon transform of the function f.

After the antipodal symmetrization of the representation (4.2.5) we obtain

$$f(x) = m_n \int_{|\omega|=1} K_+(\omega, x)\, d\omega,$$

where

$$K_+(\omega, x) = V.P. \int_{-\infty}^{\infty} \frac{1}{q}\left[\frac{\partial^{n-1}\widehat{f}(\omega, s)}{\partial s^{n-1}}\bigg|_{s=q+<\omega,x>} + \frac{\partial^{n-1}\widehat{f}(-\omega, s)}{\partial s^{n-1}}\bigg|_{s=q-<\omega,x>}\right] dq.$$

In all these formulae $V.P.$ denotes, as usual, the principal value of the integral.

It was shown in Natterer (1986) that, since the odd-order derivatives of an even function are odd functions, the relation $\widehat{f}(\omega, x) = \widehat{f}(-\omega, x)$ implies the equality

$$K_+(\omega, x) = V.P. \int_{-\infty}^{\infty} \frac{1}{q}\left[\frac{\partial^{n-1}\widehat{f}(\omega, s)}{\partial s^{n-1}}\bigg|_{s=q+<\omega,x>} - \frac{\partial^{n-1}\widehat{f}(\omega, s)}{\partial s^{n-1}}\bigg|_{s=-q+<\omega,x>}\right] dq.$$

For sufficiently regular function $\widehat{f}$, the last integrand has a removable singularity at $q = 0$. Hence, this integral does not need any regularization for the construction of the numerical algorithms for the applications needs.

On the space of the canonical line bundle $E\gamma_1$ over RP^{n-1}, consider the differential form $\Phi_x g = K_+(\tilde{\omega}, x) \cdot d\tilde{\omega}$, which is well defined because for an odd k both factors $d\omega$ and $K_+(\omega, x)$ are symmetric with respect to the antipodal involution $\omega \longleftrightarrow -\omega$ of the unit sphere. Here we denote by $d\tilde{\omega}$ the volume differential form of the projective space RP^{n-1}, which is orientable because its dimension is odd. From the definition of $\Phi_x g$, we obtain the following theorem.

Theorem 4.2.1. *If n is even, then the inversion formula for the Radon transform in $\mathbb{R}^n$ holds:*

$$f(x) = m_n \int_S \Phi_x g,$$

where S is any $(n-1)$-dimensional cycle homological to the fundamental cycle of RP^{n-1} in the fiber space $E\gamma_1$.

In the general case for any odd $k < n-1$, the differential form $\Phi_x g$ can be constructed on the Grassmann manifolds $G_{n,k,x}$ and on their unoriented analogues because the Euler cycles of all these manifolds have split normal bundles and the corresponding wedge products in the coordinate representation of $\Phi_x g$ can be arranged as in Gel'fand *et al.* (1980) for even values of dimensions R. Hence, we obtain the following theorem.

Theorem 4.2.2. *For odd k, the following inversion formula for the integral transformation J_k holds:*

$$d(Z) \cdot f(x) = m_{k+1} \int_Z \Phi_x g,$$

where Z is any k-dimensional cycle in the fiber space $E\gamma_{n-k}$.

In the particularly attractive case $k = 1$, i.e., in the tomography-type inverse problems, a finite function $f(x)$ of n real variables is to be recovered from the values of its integrals

$$g(a,b) = \int_{-\infty}^{\infty} f(b+at)\,\mathrm{d}t, \quad a,b \in \mathbb{R}^n, \qquad a \neq 0 \tag{4.2.6}$$

along the straight lines $l(a,b)$, $x = b + at$.

Since the dimension of the full projection data $E\gamma_{n-1}$ is greater than that of the space of variables $\mathbb{R}^n$, it is natural to try to reduce this data set as much as possible. For example, Gel'fand and Graev (1968) have considered n-dimensional complexes $K^n \subset E\gamma_{n-1}$ of straight lines in $\mathbb{R}^n$ such that a finite function $f(x)$ of n variables can be reconstructed from its integrals $g(a,b)$ taken along only those straight lines $l(a,b)$ which belong to K^n. It follows from (4.2.4) that all the level submanifolds of the function $g(a,b)$ (the measurements data) have split stable tangent and normal bundles in $E\gamma_{n-1}$. This is an essential restriction on the topological characteristics of these level submanifolds, in particular, for odd n the stable tangent bundles of such submanifolds admit complex self-conjugate structures (see Golubyatnikov, 1986).

It follows from the analytical properties of the Fourier transform that in order to prove the uniqueness of reconstruction of the unknown function f it is sufficient to consider a countable set of the "X-ray images" of the support supp f; each of these photographs is an $(n-1)$-dimensional data set. However, the proof of this fact is based on the consideration of an analytic continuation of some function defined on a discrete set and therefore it is not suitable for constructing algorithms which could be realized by computer programs. In the sequel the unknown functions $f(x)$ are assumed to be sufficiently differentiable.

As was shown in Kirillov (1960), if the integrals of $f(x)$ taken along all the straight lines intersecting a set $C \subset \mathbb{R}^n$ are known, then the integral of $f(x)$ taken along any straight line intersecting the convex hull of C can be determined as well. The idea of such a reduction is based on John's conditions (see Helgason, 1980), which can be immediately deduced from (4.2.6):

$$\frac{\partial^2 g}{\partial a_i \partial b_j} = \frac{\partial^2 g}{\partial a_j \partial b_i}, \qquad 1 \leq i, j \leq n. \tag{4.2.7}$$

It is easy to verify (cf. Tuy, 1983), that the function g is homogeneous with respect to the first argument:

$$g(a, c) = \frac{1}{|a|} \cdot g\left(\frac{a}{|a|}, c\right).$$

It is well known that the Fourier transform $G(\xi, b)$ of the function $g(a, b)$ with respect to the n-dimensional variable a is as regular function of its arguments at $\xi \neq 0$ as the initial unknown function $f(x)$.

It follows from the John's conditions (4.2.7) that the vectors ξ and $\mathrm{grad}_b G(\xi, b)$ are parallel. Hence, for $\xi \perp (b - c)$ we have

$$G(\xi, b) = G(\xi, c). \tag{4.2.8}$$

We recall a useful explicit formula for this function $G(\xi, b)$ in the case $n = 3$ (see Tuy, 1983).

$$G(\xi, b) = \int_0^\infty \rho \tilde{f}(\xi \cdot \rho) \exp(2\pi \mathrm{i} \rho \langle b, \xi \rangle) \, \mathrm{d}\rho. \tag{4.2.9}$$

Here $\tilde{f}$ is the Fourier transform of the unknown function f and $\langle \cdot, \cdot \rangle$ is the standard scalar product in $\mathbb{R}^3$. Similarly, in the higher-dimensional cases, if all hyperplanes containing $b \in \mathbb{R}^n$ intersect the set C, then, according to equality (4.2.8), for any $\xi \neq 0$ it is possible to find $G(\xi, b)$ if we know the integrals $g(a, c)$ for all $c \in C$ and for all nonzero vectors $a \in \mathbb{R}^n$.

Relation (4.2.8) and its analogues are used in Blagoveshchenskii (1986) and in Tuy (1983) for solution of inverse problems of integral geometry on straight lines in the Euclidean space. In particular, A. S. Blagoveshchenskii obtained an explicit formula for solution of the problem of recovery of a function with support in the cylinder $x_1^2 + \ldots + x_n^2 \leq 1$ in $\mathbb{R}^{n+1}$ if its integrals along the straight lines intersecting the $(n-1)$-dimensional sphere $x_1^2 + \ldots + x_n^2 = 1$, $x_{n+1} = 0$ are known. Here the set of these straight lines has dimension $(2n-1)$ and this is less than that of $E\gamma_n$ just by one.

For $n > 2$, it is not difficult to reduce this data set without loss of solvability of the initial inverse problem. For example, denote by S_i the unit circle centered at the origin that belongs to the two-dimensional coordinate plane $0, x_1, x_i$, where $2 \leq i \leq n+1$. Let V be the convex hull of the union of all these circles; it is a compact convex body in $\mathbb{R}^{n+1}$ with interior points. Suppose that the support of the unknown function $f(x)$ is contained in V. Then, if we know all integrals $g(a, c)$ for $|a| = 1$ and $c \in \cup S_i$, we can reconstruct the function $f(x)$ uniquely. Indeed, arguing as in Kirillov (1960), Blagoveshchenskii (1986), and Tuy (1983), it is possible to find $g(a, b)$ by equality (4.2.8) at $|a| = 1$, $b \in \cup B_i$, where B_i is a two-dimensional disk $x_1^2 + x_i^2 \leq 1$; $x_j = 0$ if $j \neq 1, i$. Step by step, we determine $g(a, b)$ at b belonging to the convex hull of two such disks B_i, then to that of three such disks, and, at last, for all $b \in V$. In such a way, we solve the inverse problem of integral geometry in $\mathbb{R}^n$ using the n-dimensional data set: the union of the circles S_i is a one-dimensional manifold and the manifold of all directions in $\mathbb{R}^n$ is $(n-1)$-dimensional.

Let us fix an arbitrary two-dimensional cross-section P^2 of the support of $f(x)$. We know the function $g(a, b)$ at $|a| = 1$ and $b \in V$. If $b \in P^2 \cap V$ and a is a unit vector parallel to P^2, the values $g(a, b)$ form the full projection data set for reconstructing the function $f(x)$ in $P^2 \cap V$ by its Radon transform in the plane P^2. Such a problem has a unique solution which can be described by explicit formulae and by computer programs. Changing P^2 we can determine $f(x)$ for all $x \in V$. It is the Nyquist frequency $N \cdot \delta x \sim \pi$ which is usually taken as the upper limit of integration in the formula (4.2.9) in computer realization of the scheme described above.

N. B. Ayupova has developed, debugged and tested programs for numerical solution of such inverse problem in $\mathbb{R}^3$. In particular, she made a series of corresponding numerical experiments of reconstruction of the characteristic functions of plane cross-sections of some 3-dimensional objects. Here the family of planes orthogonal to the axis $0, x_1$ was taken as the plane P^2.

The circles S_1 and S_2 which surround these objects were subdivided into equal arcs. Integrals of the characteristic function $f(x)$ were reconstructed for the bundles of parallel straight lines which belong to the chosen cross-section, and $f(x)$ in this cross-section was determined by the standard inversion formula of the two-dimensional Radon transform.

The reconstructed maximal value of the function $f(x)$ in these numerical experiments equals 1.016.

4.3. AN INVERSE PROBLEM FOR THE HAMILTON-JACOBI EQUATIONS

In this section we determine some sufficient conditions for the existence of a solution of the inverse problem of reconstruction of unknown Hamiltonian in the Hamilton-Jacobi equation in the case when the phase function $w(x,t)$ is known for $t = 0$ and $t = T$. This inverse problem is considered in two variants: for a domain in a Euclidean space and for a closed manifold (see Golubyatnikov, 1995c, 1997). We also find the classification of these solutions in the class of multivalued functions.

Dispersion relations are very important for studying nonlinear wave processes where the hyperbolic equations do not describe physical phenomena adequately (see, for example, Nonlinear Waves, 1974).

Here we study the problem of determination of the dispersion relation in the form of the Hamilton-Jacobi equation in the Euclidean space $\mathbb{R}^m$, provided that the phase function $w = w(x,t)$ is known at $t = 0$ and $t = T$ while the Hamiltonian $H(x, \operatorname{grad}_x w)$ has a special form: it admits m independent integrals that correspond to different conservation laws.

(a) For the Hamilton-Jacobi equation

$$w_t + H(x, \operatorname{grad}_x w) = 0 \tag{4.3.1}$$

with unknown Hamiltonian $H(x,p)$ and with the initial-terminal conditions

$$w(x,0) = a(x), \qquad w(x,T) = b(x), \tag{4.3.2}$$

where $a(x)$ and $b(x)$ are known smooth functions, we consider the inverse problem of determining two functions: $w = w(x,t)$ and $H = H(x,p)$ defined in $G \times [0,T]$ and $G \times G_1$, respectively, where $G \subseteq \mathbb{R}^m$ and $G_1 \subseteq \mathbb{R}^m$ are open convex domains.

Obviously, this problem is underdetermined. In order to obtain the uniqueness of solution of this inverse problem, we impose here some additional conditions:

(1) Let the unknown Hamiltonian $H(x,p)$ have m independent involutive integrals $f^1, f^2, \dots f^m$, $f^i = f^i(x,p)$ which are constant along the trajectories of the Hamilton system

$$\dot{x}^i = H_{p_i}, \qquad \dot{p}_i = -H_{x^i}. \tag{4.3.3}$$

For example, similar systems of integrals describe kinematic waves (see Lighthill and Witham 1955; Anikonov, 1995).

(2) There exists a canonical transformation of the domain $G \times G_1 \longrightarrow G \times G_1$ in the phase space

$$C : (x,p) \Longrightarrow (g,f)$$

under which the 2-form $\Omega = \mathrm{d}p \wedge \mathrm{d}q$ is invariant:

$$\mathrm{d}x^1 \wedge \mathrm{d}p_1 + \dots \mathrm{d}x^m \wedge \mathrm{d}p_m = \mathrm{d}f^1 \wedge \mathrm{d}g_1 + \dots \mathrm{d}f^m \wedge \mathrm{d}g_m,$$

where f^i are the integrals described above.

(3) The initial-terminal data are concordant, i.e., there exists a diffeomorphism $\psi : G \longrightarrow G$ such that

$$f^i(x, \operatorname{grad}_x a(x)) = f^i(\psi(x), \operatorname{grad}_x b(\psi(x))), \quad i = 1, \dots m.$$

Since the transformation $C : (x,p) \Longrightarrow (g,f)$ is canonical, the original equation (4.3.1) and the initial-terminal conditions (4.3.2) in the new coordinates (g,f) have the form

$$w_t + H(x(g,f), \operatorname{grad}_x w) = 0,$$

$$w(x(g,f),0) = a(x(g,f)), \qquad w(x(g,f),T) = b(x(g,f)).$$

In these coordinates the Hamilton system (4.3.3) becomes simpler:

$$\dot{g}_i = -H_{f^i}, \qquad \dot{f}^i = H_{g_i} = 0 \tag{4.3.4}$$

because f^i are integrals of the system (4.3.3). Hence, the Hamiltonian H does not depend on the variables g_i dual to the integrals f^i and we can integrate the Hamilton system in these angle-action variables, as in Arnol'd (1978).

The points of the phase space $G \times G_1$

$$(g(x, \operatorname{grad}_x a(x)), f(x, \operatorname{grad}_x a(x)))$$

and

$$(g(\psi(x), \operatorname{grad}_x b(\psi(x))), f(\psi(x), \operatorname{grad}_x b(\psi(x))))$$

belong to the same trajectory of the Hamilton system (4.3.4) for any $x \in G$. Hence, on any such trajectory $H_{f^i} = \text{const}$ the coordinates g_i of the points depend on t linearly:

$$g(\psi(x), \operatorname{grad}_x b(\psi(x))) - g(x, \operatorname{grad}_x a(x)) = T \cdot \operatorname{grad}_f H.$$

This yields the explicit formula for the group velocity $\operatorname{grad}_f H$ which allows to express the function $g(x, p)$ in terms of t along the trajectories of the system (4.3.4):

$$g(x, p) = \left(1 - \frac{t}{T}\right) \cdot g(x, \operatorname{grad}_x a(x)) + \frac{t}{T} \cdot g(\psi(x), \operatorname{grad}_x b(\psi(x))). \quad (4.3.5)$$

(4) Equation (4.3.5) defines a nonsingular change of variables in the domain $G \times G_1$ for all $t \in [0, T]$.

Theorem 4.3.1. *Under conditions* **(1)–(4)** *the inverse problem* (4.3.1), (4.3.2) *has a unique solution* $w(x, t), H(x, p)$ *defined in* $G \times [0, T]$ *and* $G \times G_1$, *respectively.*

Proof. We use the canonical transformation inverse to C in order to find the gradient $\operatorname{grad}_x w = p(g, f)$, where f and g are the same as in (4.3.5). Then the initial-terminal conditions uniquely determine the phase function w, which allows us to find the unknown Hamiltonian H from (4.3.1). □

We shall derive some corollaries of Theorem 4.3.1. For this purpose, we make other assumptions which guarantee that conditions **(2)**, **(3)** of this theorem are satisfied.

(5) The Hamiltonian H is independent of the space variables x, and the gradients $\operatorname{grad}_x a$, $\operatorname{grad}_x b : G \longrightarrow G_1$ are diffeomorphisms.

The Hamilton systems with such Hamiltonians describe nonlinear wave propagation in homogeneous media (see Nonlinear Waves, 1974). That is why their Hamiltonians usually are called homogeneous. Here

$H_{x^i} = -p^i = 0$, i. e., the gradient of the wave function w, the wave vector, and the group velocity H_{p^i}, which determines the direction of the energy flow, are constant along the trajectories of the system (4.3.3). In this case all these trajectories are straight lines and the canonical transformation C is the identical one.

If condition **(5)** is satisfied, Theorem 4.3.1 implies

$$\operatorname{grad}_x w(x^1 \dots x^m, t) = A[x - t \cdot \operatorname{grad}_p H],$$

where the arguments in the gradient of the Hamiltonian H have the form $p = \operatorname{grad}_x w$, i.e., $p_i = w_{x^i}$ and the vector-function A is defined by $A(y^1, \dots y^m) = \operatorname{grad}_y a(y^1, \dots y^m)$. In a similar way we shall define the vector-function $B(y^1, \dots y^m) = \operatorname{grad}_y b(y^1, \dots y^m)$.

Equation (4.3.5) yields

$$\operatorname{grad}_p H(p_1, \dots p_m) = \frac{1}{T}[B^{-1}(p_1, \dots p_m) - A^{-1}(p_1, \dots p_m)].$$

For the case of homogeneous Hamiltonians, this equation was considered by Yu. E. Anikonov.

Following the structure of the well known formula of the partition of a segment in a given proportion, we rewrite (4.3.5) in the more symmetric form

$$x = (1 - \tau) \cdot A^{-1}(\operatorname{grad}_x w) + \tau \cdot B^{-1}(\operatorname{grad}_x w) = F(p), \tag{4.3.6}$$

and verify condition **(4)**, i. e., whether equation (4.3.6) has a unique solution $\operatorname{grad}_x w = \Phi(x, t)$. Here $\tau = t/T$, $0 \le \tau \le 1$.

First, we consider the simplest case of quadratic functions $a(x)$ and $b(x)$ defined in the whole Euclidean space $\mathbb{R}^m$. Their gradients are linear vector-functions: $\operatorname{grad}_x a = A \cdot x$ and $\operatorname{grad}_x b = B \cdot x$, where A and B denote the corresponding $m \times m$-matrices. Multiplying equation (4.3.6) by A, we obtain

$$A \cdot x = [(1 - \tau) \cdot E + \tau \cdot A \cdot B^{-1}](\operatorname{grad}_x w). \tag{4.3.7}$$

Here E denotes the unit $m \times m$-matrix. We can solve this equation for $\operatorname{grad}_x w$ at any $\tau \in [0, 1]$ if and only if in the right-hand side of (4.3.7) the gradient $\operatorname{grad}_x w$ is multiplied by a regular matrix.

Corollary 4.3.1. If the inverse problem (4.3.1), (4.3.2) has a homogeneous Hamiltonian $H(x, p)$ and satisfies condition **(5)** for $G = G_1 = \mathbb{R}^m$, then the functions $w(x, t)$ and $H(x, p)$ are uniquely determined in $\mathbb{R}^m \times [0, T]$

and $\mathbb{R}^{2m}$, respectively, if and only if the matrix $A \cdot B^{-1}$ has no negative eigenvalues.

Similarly, we can describe the solvability conditions for (4.3.6) in the case of quadratic functions a and b defined in the open half-space $G \subset \mathbb{R}^m$ bounded by the hyperspace orthogonal to a common eigenvector of the matrices A and B that corresponds to their positive eigenvalues.

Now, let $a(x)$ and $b(x)$ be arbitrary functions whose gradients determine diffeomorphisms $\operatorname{grad}_x a$, $\operatorname{grad}_x b : G \longrightarrow G_1$.

Let us suppose that equation (4.3.6) is not uniquely solvable, i. e., $F(p_1) = F(p_2)$ for some $p_1 \neq p_2$. Denote by $J_A^{-1}(p)$ and $J_B^{-1}(p)$ the Jacobi matrices of the diffeomorphisms $\operatorname{grad}_x a$ and $\operatorname{grad}_x b$, respectively. Using the notation $l = p_1 - p_2 \neq 0$, we define the operators $T_A(p_2, l)$ and $T_B(p_2, l)$ with the help of the Newton–Leibnitz formula:

$$A^{-1}(p_1) - A^{-1}(p_2) = \int_0^1 J_A^{-1}(p_2 + l \cdot t) \cdot l \, \mathrm{d}t = T_A(p_2, l) \cdot l,$$

$$B^{-1}(p_1) - B^{-1}(p_2) = \int_0^1 J_B^{-1}(p_2 + l \cdot t) \cdot l \, \mathrm{d}t = T_B(p_2, l) \cdot l.$$

Here $J^{-1} \cdot l$ is the product of the matrix J^{-1} and the vector l.

Since $F(p_1) = F(p_2)$,

$$[(1 - \tau) \cdot T_A(p_2, l) + \tau \cdot T_B(p_2, l)] \cdot l = 0, \tag{4.3.8}$$

or, if $0 \neq \tau \neq 1$,

$$\Big[E + \frac{\tau}{1 - \tau}(T_A^{-1}(p_2, l) \cdot T_B(p_2, l))\Big] \cdot l = 0.$$

Consequently, if the operator $T_A^{-1}(p_2, l) \cdot T_B(p_2, l)$ exists and has no negative eigenvalues, the gradient $\operatorname{grad}_x w$ is uniquely determined by equation (4.3.6).

In particular, if $a(x)$ and $b(x)$ are strictly convex functions defined on the space $\mathbb{R}^m$, then the matrices $J_A^{-1}(p)$ and $J_B^{-1}(p)$ are positive definite because they are inverse to the Hesse matrices of the initial-terminal values $a(x)$ and $b(x)$ of the phase function.

Consider the scalar products of equation (4.3.8) by the vector l:

$$(1 - \tau) \cdot \langle T_A(p_2, l) \cdot l, l \rangle + \tau \cdot \langle T_B(p_2, l) \cdot l, l \rangle = 0.$$

On the other hand,

$$\langle T_A(p_2,l)\cdot l,l\rangle = \int_0^1 \langle J_A^{-1}(p_2+l\cdot t)\cdot l,l\rangle\,\mathrm{d}t > 0,$$

$$\langle T_B(p_2,l)\cdot l,l\rangle = \int_0^1 \langle J_B^{-1}(p_2+l\cdot t)\cdot l,l\rangle\,\mathrm{d}t > 0.$$

In our considerations, τ and $(1-\tau)$ are positive, J_A^{-1} and J_B^{-1} are positive definite. Therefore, these two inequalities lead to a contradiction, and we obtain the following

Corollary 4.3.2. If the inverse problem (4.3.1)–(4.3.2) has homogeneous Hamiltonian $H(x,p)$ and strictly convex functions a and b satisfy **(5)** for $G = G_1 = \mathbb{R}^m$, then the functions w and H are uniquely determined in $\mathbb{R}^m \times [0,T]$ and $\mathbb{R}^{2m}$, respectively.

(b) Now, we shall consider this inverse problem in the case when the phase function and the Hamiltonian are defined on a closed manifold. Namely, let M^m be a closed, compact, connected, simply connected, smooth m-dimensional manifold with a fixed orientation. Let $\pi : T^*M^m \longrightarrow M^m$ be its cotangent bundle with canonical symplectic structure determined by the 2-form $\Omega = \mathrm{d}p \wedge \mathrm{d}x$. We consider the inverse problem of determining two unknown functions $w(x,t)$ and $H(x,p)$ defined on the cylinder $M^m \times [0,1]$ and in some domain of the phase space T^*M^m, respectively, provided that the phase function of the wave process $w(x,t)$ is a solution of the Hamilton–Jacobi equation (4.3.1) with unknown Hamiltonian $H(x,p)$ and satisfies the initial-terminal conditions (4.3.2), where $a(x)$ and $b(x)$ are known smooth functions on the manifold M^m.

Clearly, the problem (4.3.1)–(4.3.2) is strongly underdetermined as in the case of an open domain in a Euclidean space. Indeed, it is usually impossible to determine a function of $m+1$ variables and a function of $2m$ variables uniquely from two known functions of m variables. As above, we shall impose some additional conditions on the initial-terminal data in order to minimize the nonuniqueness as much as possible.

Denote by $s_a, s_b : M \longrightarrow T^*M^m$ the gradient sections of the cotangent bundle T^*M^m that relate each point $x \in M^m$ to the values of the gradients $\operatorname{grad}_x a(x)$ and $\operatorname{grad}_x b(x)$, respectively, and denote by

$$\Gamma_a = \{(x,p) \mid \operatorname{grad}_x a = p\}, \qquad \Gamma_b = \{(x,p) \mid \operatorname{grad}_x b = p\}$$

the graphs of these gradients.

(6) Let the unknown Hamiltonian $H(x,p)$ have m independent involutive integrals $f^1, f^2, \dots f^m$, $f^i = f^i(x,p)$ and let the corresponding moment map

$$\Phi = (f^1, \dots f^m) : T^*M^m \longrightarrow R^m$$

defined by these integrals be proper, i.e., it maps noncompact sets to noncompact sets.

According to Liouville's theorem (see, for example, Arnol'd, 1978), in this case the connected components of the preimages of the regular values of Φ are diffeomorphic to the m-dimensional torus T^m and the skew gradients sgrad $f^1, \dots,$ sgrad f^m of these integrals determine the parallelization of these tori, which are called nonsingular or Liouville's tori.

(7) Following Bott (1954), we shall assume that all the critical points of Φ are nondegenerate, i. e., the set C_Φ of these critical points is decomposed into the union of submanifolds and at each point $x \in C_\Phi$ the differential $\mathrm{d}\Phi$ is nondegenerate in the directions transversal to C_Φ at x; furthermore, the relation corank $\mathrm{d}\Phi > 1$ holds at all critical points of the map Φ.

If conditions **(6)**, **(7)** are satisfied, then, using the skew gradients of the integrals, we can associate with Φ the action of T^m, considered as an abelian group, on the phase space T^*M^m :

$$\mu : T^m \times T^*M^m \longrightarrow T^*M^m.$$

In this case, the connected component of the inverse image of the irregular values of Φ is diffeomorphic to the tori $T^{(m-k)}$, $m \geq k > 0$, of lower dimensions, obtained by factorization of the m-dimensional torus by the stabilizers of the critical points forming these singular tori $T^{(m-k)}$.

Our further constructions will proceed in some T^m-invariant bounded domain $D \subset T^*M$ which contains the graphs Γ_a and Γ_b.

(8) We shall assume that the initial-terminal conditions (4.3.2) are in general position with the moment map Φ and are concordant, i. e.,

(i) the graphs Γ_a and Γ_b and the set of the critical points of Φ are in general position;

(ii) for every singular or nonsingular torus T, the intersections of T with the graphs Γ_a and Γ_b are the translates of each other under some parallel translation $g(T)$ in the angular coordinates of this torus.

In particular, the condition (ii) is satisfied if each of these intersections consists of a single point or is empty, and the condition (i) implies that the dimensions of the intersections of Γ_a and Γ_b with the set of critical points Φ do not exceed $(m-3)$ and hence their complements in Γ_a and Γ_b are simply connected (see Montgomery *et al.*, 1956; Guillemin and Sternberg, 1982).

Therefore, every two Liouville's tori intersecting Γ_a and Γ_b can be joined by a smooth one-parameter family of nonsingular tori which also intersect the graphs of the gradients of functions a and b. In the sequel, unless otherwise stipulated, we shall consider only those tori, singular or nonsingular, whose intersections with these graphs are nonempty.

Note that under our assumptions we can reconstruct the values of the unknown Hamiltonian $H(x,p)$ only on the union of the tori which are the μ-orbits of the points of Γ_a and Γ_b. We have no data for determination of $H(x,p)$ outside this union.

The proper moment map Φ admits an extension to the map of one-point compactifications:

$$\phi : MT^*M^m \longrightarrow S^m.$$

Here the Thom space of the cotangent bundle over M^m mapped into the m-dimensional sphere. Denote $\phi^*(1)$ by $kU \in H^m(MT^*M^m)$, where U is the integer Thom class of the cotangent bundle, k is an integer, $1 \in H^m(S^m)$ is the generator of the integer cohomology group. As was shown in Golubyatnikov (1986),

$$kU \cup kU = \phi^*(1 \cup 1) = 0 \in H^{2m}(MT^*M^m) \approx Z.$$

Hence, if $k \neq 0$ then the product $U \cup U$ and the Euler characteristic of M^m vanish; and vice versa: if $U \cup U \neq 0$ then the coefficient k is zero.

Therefore, the product $kU \cup U$ vanishes in all cases. Thus, the dual homology classes, i. e., every integral manifold (a Liouville's torus T) and every cycle homological to a section (the gradient graph of a smooth function) have zero intersection index. Hence, the typical nonempty intersections $\Gamma_a \cap T$ and $\Gamma_b \cap T$ consist of even numbers of points with intersection indices of opposite signs.

For some nonsingular torus T_0, choose a tangent vector field $v(T_0)$ which has constant components in the angular coordinates and such that its integral trajectories realize the parallel translation $g(T_0)$ from $\Gamma_a \cap T_0$ to $\Gamma_b \cap T_0$ when t varies from 0 to 1. It is obvious that all such vector fields are classified by the fundamental group of the m-dimensional torus T_0. According to Liouville's theorem, this vector field $v(T_0)$ can be extended to some neighborhood of T_0 so that its restriction $v(T)$ to any other nonsingular torus T (which still intersects Γ_a and Γ_b) is constant in the angular coordinates on T and likewise $v(T_0)$ is tangent to the trajectories of the parallel translation $g(T)$.

The compactness of the closure of D implies that D contains finitely many critical manifolds of the moment map Φ, and the μ-orbits of these points of these manifolds are singular tori diffeomorphic to $T^{(m-k)} = T^m/T^k$. Therefore, on the union of all nonsingular tori intersecting the graphs of the gradients of the initial-terminal data a and b, we can construct a vector field v whose restriction to every such torus T coincides with $v(T)$ and whose restrictions to the set of singular tori determine the parallel translation mentioned in the condition (ii). Connectedness and simple connectedness of the set of singular tori imply that the limit values of v are well defined on singular tori as well.

We introduce some notation: given $x \in M^m$, let $T(x) \subset T^*M$ be the μ-orbit of the point $s_a(x) = (x, \operatorname{grad}_x a(x))$; let $\gamma(x,t)$ be a point on the trajectory of the vector field $v(T(x))$ which starts from $s_a(x)$; and let $\gamma_t : M^m \longrightarrow T^*M^m$ be a map such that $\gamma_t(x) = \gamma(x,t)$, $0 \le t \le 1$. Clearly, for all such t the so-constructed γ_t is an embedding. Let $\psi_t(x) = \pi \circ \gamma_t(x)$ be the projection of the trajectory $\gamma(x,t)$ to the configuration manifold M^m; by definitions one has $\psi_0(x) = x$, $\psi_1(x) = \pi \circ g(T(x)) \circ s_a(x)$.

Lemma 4.3.1. *For all $t \in [0,1]$ the image $\gamma_t(M)$ is a Lagrangian submanifold in the phase space and the map $\psi_t : M \longrightarrow M$ has degree one.*

Proof. Calculate the value of the 2-form Ω on any pair of vectors r_t and s_t tangent to $\gamma_t(M)$. In the angle-action coordinates, these vectors can be expressed as linear combinations of the corresponding vectors tangent to $\gamma_0(M) = \Gamma_a$ and to $\gamma_1(M) = \Gamma_b$ with constant coefficients of the action coordinates and linear (in t) coefficients of the angular coordinates. Hence, $\Omega(r_t, s_t)$ depends linearly on t as well. Since $\gamma_0(M)$ and $\gamma_1(M)$ are Lagrangian submanifolds in $T^*(M)$, the form $\Omega(r_t, s_t)$ vanishes at $t = 0$ and $t = 1$; therefore, it vanishes for all values of t.

The second part of the statement follows from the fact that the family of mappings $\psi_t : M^m \longrightarrow M^m$ is a smooth homotopy of the identity diffeomorphism ψ_0 because of the smoothness of the vector field v. □

For all $t \in [0,1]$, the above Lagrangian manifolds $\gamma_t(M)$ are the gradient graphs $\operatorname{grad}_x w$ of some $w(x,t)$ (in general, a multivalued function with singularities) which is a solution to the problem (4.3.1), (4.3.2). This implies the following theorem.

Theorem 4.3.2. *If conditions* **(6)–(8)** *hold, then the inverse problem* (4.3.1), (4.3.2) *has solutions in the class of multivalued functions with singularities, and these solutions are classified by the fundamental group of an* m*-dimensional torus.*

The theory of multivalued functions and functionals has been studied in many publications (see, for example, Novikov, 1982). Here we are interested in conditions under which the phase function $w(x,t)$ is single valued and has no singularities, and the manifolds $\gamma_t(M)$ for all above indicated t are projected onto M^m diffeomorphically. In this case, knowing the gradient $\text{grad}_x w$, we can find the function w up to a summand which depends only on t, but the initial-terminal data (4.3.2) determine this summand uniquely. Hence, the next theorem is valid:

Theorem 4.3.3. *If under the assumptions of Theorem 4.3.2 the differential of the mapping* $\psi_t : M^m \longrightarrow M^m$ *is nondegenerate for all* $t \in [0,1]$ *and for all points* $x \in M$, *then the inverse problem* (4.3.1), (4.3.2) *has a smooth single-valued solution without singularities.*

Proof. It is sufficient to verify that, under the condition of nondegeneracy of the differential $d\psi_t$, the Lagrangian manifold $\gamma_t(M)$ is projected onto M^m diffeomorphically.

Indeed, as was shown in Lemma 4.3.1, the degree of ψ_t equals one. Let the mapping ψ_t take two different points into one point x_0 for some t. By Sard's theorem, without loss of generality we may assume x_0 to be a regular value of ψ_t. Since the sum of degrees of this mapping over all preimages of x_0 at which the degree of ψ_t equals one, there are points x_+ and x_- in this preimage at which the degree of ψ_t equals $+1$ and -1, respectively. As far as M^m is connected, on every curve joining these points x_+ and x_- there are points where the differential of ψ_t degenerates, which contradicts the assumption of the theorem. □

It is seen from these arguments that the condition of nondegeneracy of $d\psi_t$ could be relaxed admitting a discrete set of points where the differential degenerates. In these points the singe-valued solution of the original inverse problem will have singularities.

As follows from the theorem on noncommutative integration of Hamilton systems (Fomenko, 1995; Fomenko and Mishchenko, 1981), Theorems 4.3.2 and 4.3.3 remain valid, with the corresponding correction of dimensions, if the integrals $f^1, f^2, \ldots$ are not in involution but constitute a maximal linear finite-dimensional algebra on T^*M^m.

4.4. INVERSE PROBLEMS FOR ONE CLASS OF THE TOMOGRAPHY-TYPE EVOLUTION EQUATIONS

This section is devoted to continuation of the study of solutions to the multidimensional evolution equation

$$w_t = \mathbf{A}\, w + \lambda(x) f(t) \tag{4.4.1}$$

with initial and terminal conditions (Input-Output data)

$$w|_{t=a} = w_a(x); \quad w|_{t=b} = w_b(x), \tag{4.4.2}$$

which was started in Anikonov (1994), Anikonov and Vishnevskii (1996). Here $x = (x^1, \ldots, x^n) \in D \subseteq \mathbb{R}^n$, $w_a(x)$ and $w_b(x)$ are unknown functions, $w(x,t)$ is smooth in t, $f(t)$ is continuous, $a \le t \le b$, $a < b$, and $\mathbf{A}$ is a linear operator that acts with respect to the space variables and has the real symbol $A_0(\xi)$: $\mathbf{A}\, \mathrm{e}^{\mathrm{i}\xi x} = A_0(\xi)\mathrm{e}^{\mathrm{i}\xi x}$, where $\xi \in \mathbb{R}^n$. Most results of this section were obtained in the joint papers Ayupova and Golubyatnikov (1997, 1998). The study of similar inverse problems is also described in Prilepko (1992).

In Anikonov (1994), Anikonov and Vishnevskii (1996), the explicit formal solutions to the inverse problem of finding functions $\mathcal{W}(x,t)$ and $\Lambda(x)$ satisfying (4.4.1), (4.4.2) were constructed and, under the assumption that $|f(t)| > 0$ for all $t \in [a,b]$ conditions were obtained for these formal solutions to be well defined.

The general outline of these arguments was as follows:

A) On carrying out the Fourier transform in space variables, it becomes possible to solve the evolution equation explicitly by making use of the semigroup generated by $\mathbf{A}$ (see Orlovskii, 1990; Tikhonov and Eidel'man, 1994).

B) In order to solve the original inverse problem, the inverse Fourier transform $\mathcal{F}^{-1}$ is applied to the obtained explicit inversion formulae for $\widehat{w}(\xi,t)$ and $\widehat{\lambda}(\xi)$. This gives rise to the problem of regularity of images of these transforms and the problem of convergence of the integrals and series involved.

The general structure of the explicit formulae for these solutions corresponds to the well-known partition of a segment $[a,b]$ in a given proportion $(t-a):(b-t)$, just like in Section 4.3.

So, the problem of determination of these two unknown functions $w(x,t)$ and $\lambda(x)$ from the initial-terminal data (4.4.2) has a natural tomographic interpretation.

Following Anikonov (1994), we say that the formal solutions $\widehat{w}(\xi,t)$ and $\widehat{\lambda}(\xi)$ are well defined and that they give solutions to the inverse problem (4.4.1), (4.4.2) if the functions $\mathcal{F}^{-1}\,\widehat{w}(\xi,t)$ and $\mathcal{F}^{-1}\widehat{\lambda}(\xi)$ belong to the specified function spaces, namely, in Theorem 4.4.2 they should belong to the space of infinitely differentiable rapidly decreasing functions and in Theorem 4.4.1 to the spaces $\mathbf{W}_2^m(D)$ and $\mathbf{W}_2^{m-2}(D)$, etc.

In the beginning of this section we show that such correctness holds in the one-dimenional case for a wider class of continuous functions f; in the last subsection we consider an analogous inverse problem for a system of evolution equations similar to (4.4.1).

(a) Let $D \subset \mathbb{R}^n$ be a bounded domain with smooth boundary; let $\mathbf{A}$ be an elliptic operator of the second order with smooth coefficients:

$$\mathbf{A} = \sum_{i,j=1}^{n} \frac{\partial}{\partial x^i}\Big(a_{i,j}(x)\frac{\partial}{\partial x^j}\Big) + a(x),$$

and suppose that the solution to (4.4.1), as in Anikonov and Vishnevskii (1996), satisfies a certain boundary-value condition, for instance, $\Gamma w = 0$, where

$$\Gamma = \alpha_1\Bigg(\sum_{i,j=1}^{n} a_{i,j}(x)\frac{\partial}{\partial x^i}\cos(N, x^i) + \sigma(x)\Bigg) + \alpha_0, \tag{4.4.3}$$

$x \in \partial D$, N is the unit normal to ∂D, $\alpha_1 \geq 0$, and $\alpha_1^2 + \alpha_0^2 > 0$.

It is well known (see Ladyzhenskaya and Ural'ceva 1968, Chapter 3) that, under a condition of the form (4.4.3), the spectral problem $\mathbf{A}T = \lambda T$ has discrete spectrum with unique limit point which is at minus infinity. Denote by $T_k(x)$, λ_k, $k = 1, 2, \ldots$, the eigenfunctions and eigenvalues of this spectral problem. For the sake of simplicity, we also introduce the notation

$$Z_k(\alpha, \beta) = \int_{\alpha}^{\beta} f(p)\mathrm{e}^{-\lambda_k p}\,\mathrm{d}p, \qquad [\alpha, \beta] \subseteq [a, b].$$

Denote by J the set of all indices k such that $Z_k(a, b) = 0$. For such k, the function $\gamma_k(t) = \mathrm{e}^{\lambda_k t} Z_k(a, t)$ satisfies the relation $\mathrm{d}\gamma_k/\mathrm{d}t - \lambda_k\gamma_k = f(t)$ and vanishes at the endpoints of $[a, b]$.

Since $\lambda_k \to -\infty$ as $k \to \infty$, it follows that for all real $p > q$ there exists a k_0 such that the following inequalities hold for all $k > k_0$:

$$\lambda_k(p - q) < -\ln 2; \quad \mathrm{e}^{-\lambda_k p} > 2\mathrm{e}^{-\lambda_k q}; \quad \mathrm{e}^{-\lambda_k p} - \mathrm{e}^{-\lambda_k q} > \mathrm{e}^{-\lambda_k p}/2. \tag{4.4.4}$$

Expand the initial and terminal conditions (4.4.2) into series in eigenfunctions $T_k(x)$. As is noted in Anikonov and Vishnevskii (1996), if $w_a(x)$

and $w_b(x)$ are in $\mathbf{W}_2^m(D)$, then $T_k(x) \in \mathbf{W}_2^m(D)$ for all k and, in this case, the series

$$w_a(x) = \sum_{k=1}^{\infty} a_k T_k(x), \quad w_b(x) = \sum_{k=1}^{\infty} b_k T_k(x) \tag{4.4.5}$$

converge in $\mathbf{W}_2^m(D)$.

We write the solution to the problem (4.4.1), (4.4.2) obtained in Anikonov and Vishnevskii (1996) in a modified form:

$$\mathcal{W}(x,t) = \sum_{k \notin J} T_k(x) h_k(t) \tag{4.4.6}$$

and

$$\Lambda(x) = \sum_{k \notin J} \frac{b_k \mathrm{e}^{-\lambda_k b} - a_k \mathrm{e}^{-\lambda_k a}}{Z_k(a,b)} T_k(x), \tag{4.4.7}$$

where

$$h_k(t) = \frac{a_k \mathrm{e}^{\lambda_k (t-a)} Z_k(t,b) + b_k \mathrm{e}^{\lambda_k (t-b)} Z_k(a,t)}{Z_k(a,b)}$$

and the coefficients a_k and b_k are given by (4.4.5).

Theorem 4.4.1. *1) Let $f(t)$ be a continuous function on $[a,b]$, $f(b) \neq 0$, and suppose that for all $k \in J$ we have $a_k = b_k = 0$. Then the set J is finite and the functions*

$$w(x,t) = \mathcal{W}(x,t) + \sum_{k \in J} c_k \gamma_k(t) T_k(x) \tag{4.4.8}$$

and

$$\lambda(x) = \Lambda(x) + \sum_{k \in J} c_k T_k(x) \tag{4.4.9}$$

determine a formal solution to (4.4.1), (4.4.2) for arbitrary constants c_k.

2) Furthermore, if the initial and terminal data $w_a(x)$ and $w_b(x)$ belong to the space $\mathbf{W}_2^m(D)$ with $m > 2$, then the series (4.4.8) converges in $\mathbf{W}_2^m(D)$ for all $t \in [a,b]$ and the series (4.4.9) converges in $\mathbf{W}_2^{m-2}(D)$.

Note that possible nonuniqueness of a solution to (4.4.1), (4.4.2) appearing in formulae (4.4.8) and (4.4.9) was earlier established in Orlovskii (1990).

Proof. For definiteness, assume that $f(t) > 0$ on $(c,b]$, where $a < c < b$, and let $c < c_1 < b$. Introduce the following notation:

$$f_2 = \inf_{t \in [c_1,b]} f(t) > 0; \quad f_3 = \inf_{t \in [a,c]} f(t).$$

Following the argument in Anikonov and Vishnevskii (1996), we take a summand of (4.4.6) and estimate its denominator by putting $f_1 = \sup_{t\in[a,b]} |f(t)|$. We have

$$Z_k(a,b) = \int_a^c f(\tau)e^{-\tau\lambda_k}\,d\tau + \int_c^{c_1} f(\tau)e^{-\tau\lambda_k}\,d\tau + \int_{c_1}^b f(\tau)e^{-\tau\lambda_k}\,d\tau. \quad (4.4.10)$$

The second term of this sum is positive and the third term admits the following estimate

$$\int_{c_1}^b f(\tau)e^{-\tau\lambda_k}\,d\tau \geq \frac{f_2}{-\lambda_k}\left(e^{-\lambda_k b} - e^{-\lambda_k c_1}\right).$$

Consider two cases:

(i) If the first summand in (4.4.10) is positive, then

$$Z_k(a,b) > \frac{f_2}{-\lambda_k}\left(e^{-\lambda_k b} - e^{-\lambda_k c_1}\right) > 0.$$

(ii) If the first summand in (4.4.10) is negative, then it is greater than

$$\frac{f_3}{-\lambda_k}\left(e^{-\lambda_k c} - e^{-\lambda_k a}\right), \quad f_3 < 0,$$

which implies

$$\begin{aligned} Z_k(a,b) &> \frac{f_2}{-\lambda_k}\left(e^{-\lambda_k b} - e^{-\lambda_k c_1}\right) - \frac{-f_3}{-\lambda_k}\left(e^{-\lambda_k c} - e^{-\lambda_k a}\right) \\ &> \frac{f_2}{-\lambda_k}\left(e^{-\lambda_k b} - e^{-\lambda_k c_1}\right) - \frac{-f_3}{-\lambda_k}e^{-\lambda_k c}. \end{aligned}$$

For k sufficiently large such that $\lambda_k(b - c_1) < -\ln 2$, we have

$$\left(e^{-\lambda_k b} - e^{-\lambda_k c_1}\right) > e^{-\lambda_k b}/2$$

and then

$$Z_k(a,b) > \frac{f_2}{-2\lambda_k}e^{-\lambda_k b} - \frac{-f_3}{-\lambda_k}e^{-\lambda_k c} > 0.$$

In the case (i), the factor of b_k in (4.4.6) is estimated as follows:

$$\left|\frac{e^{\lambda_k(t-b)}\int_a^t f(\tau)e^{-\tau\lambda_k}\,d\tau}{\int_a^b f(\tau)e^{-\tau\lambda_k}\,d\tau}\right| \le \frac{e^{\lambda_k(t-b)}f_1(e^{-\lambda_k t}-e^{-\lambda_k a})}{f_2(e^{-\lambda_k b}-e^{-\lambda_k c_1})}$$

$$= \frac{f_1(1-e^{\lambda_k(t-a)})}{f_2(1-e^{\lambda_k(b-c_1)})} < \frac{f_1/f_2}{1-e^{\lambda_k(b-c_1)}},$$

which is less than $2f_1/f_2$ for $\lambda_k(b-c_1) < -\ln 2$.

In the case (ii), the factor of b_k is estimated in the following way:

$$\left|\frac{e^{\lambda_k(t-b)}\int_a^t f(\tau)e^{-\tau\lambda_k}\,d\tau}{\int_a^b f(\tau)e^{-\tau\lambda_k}\,d\tau}\right| \le \frac{e^{\lambda_k(t-b)}f_1(e^{-\lambda_k t}-e^{-\lambda_k a})}{((f_2/2)\,e^{-\lambda_k b}-(-f_3)e^{-\lambda_k c})}$$

$$= \frac{f_1(1-e^{\lambda_k(t-a)})}{(f_2/2)-(-f_3)e^{\lambda_k(b-c)}} < \frac{2f_1/f_2}{1-(-(2f_3/f_2))e^{\lambda_k(b-c)}},$$

which is less than $4f_1/f_2 = \widetilde{K} > 0$ for $\lambda_k(b-c) < -\ln(-4f_3/f_2)$.

We now estimate the factor of a_k in (4.4.6) for k sufficiently large.

Case (i):

$$\left|\frac{e^{\lambda_k(t-a)}\int_t^b f(\tau)e^{-\tau\lambda_k}\,d\tau}{\int_a^b f(\tau)e^{-\tau\lambda_k}\,d\tau}\right| \le \frac{e^{\lambda_k(t-a)}f_1(e^{-\lambda_k b}-e^{-\lambda_k t})}{f_2(e^{-\lambda_k b}-e^{-\lambda_k c_1})} < \frac{f_1/f_2}{1-e^{-\lambda_k(b-c_1)}},$$

which is less than $2f_1/f_2$ for $\lambda_k(b-c_1) < -\ln 2$.

In the case (ii), we have:

$$\left|\frac{e^{\lambda_k(t-a)}\int_t^b f(\tau)e^{-\tau\lambda_k}\,d\tau}{\int_a^b f(\tau)e^{-\tau\lambda_k}\,d\tau}\right| \le \frac{f_1(e^{\lambda_k(t-a)}-e^{\lambda_k(b-a)})}{f_2(1-(-(2f_3/f_2))e^{\lambda_k(b-c)})/2}$$

$$< \frac{2f_1/f_2}{1-(-(2f_3/f_2))e^{\lambda_k(b-c)}},$$

which is less than $4f_1/f_2 = \widetilde{K}$ for $\lambda_k(b-c) < -\ln(-4f_3/f_2)$.

Therefore, for k sufficiently large,

$$|w_k(x,t)| \le \widetilde{K}(|a_k| + |b_k|),$$

which implies the required convergence of (4.4.6).

From the above estimates it follows that $Z_k(a,b) > 0$ for k sufficiently large, which means that the set J is finite.

We now verify the convergence of (4.4.7).

By the definition of $\Lambda(x)$, the coefficients of $T_k(x)$ in (4.4.7) can be estimated in modulus by

$$\frac{|b_k|\,\mathrm{e}^{-\lambda_k b} + |a_k|\,\mathrm{e}^{-\lambda_k a}}{\int\limits_a^b f(\tau)\mathrm{e}^{-\tau\lambda_k}\,\mathrm{d}\tau} = \frac{|b_k|\,\mathrm{e}^{-\lambda_k b} + |a_k|\,\mathrm{e}^{-\lambda_k a}}{Z_k(a,b)}.$$

In the case (i), for k sufficiently large, the above value is less than

$$\frac{|b_k|\,\mathrm{e}^{-\lambda_k b} + |a_k|\,\mathrm{e}^{-\lambda_k a}}{(f_2/-\lambda_k)(\mathrm{e}^{-\lambda_k b} - \mathrm{e}^{-\lambda_k c_1})} = \frac{|\lambda_k|\,(\,|b_k| + |a_k|\,\mathrm{e}^{\lambda_k(b-a)})}{f_2(1 - \mathrm{e}^{\lambda_k(b-c_1)})}$$

and in the case (ii) it is less than

$$\frac{|b_k|\,\mathrm{e}^{-\lambda_k b} + |a_k|\,\mathrm{e}^{-\lambda_k a}}{(f_2/(-2\lambda_k))\mathrm{e}^{-\lambda_k b} - (-f_3)/(-\lambda_k)\mathrm{e}^{-\lambda_k c}} = \frac{2\,|\lambda_k|\,(\,|b_k| + |a_k|\,\mathrm{e}^{\lambda_k(b-a)})}{f_2(1 - 2(-f_3)\mathrm{e}^{\lambda_k(b-c)})}.$$

For k sufficiently large, both right-hand sides are less than $C\,|\lambda_k|\,(\,|b_k|+|a_k|\,)$, where C is some positive constant, and thus the statement in the second part of Theorem 4.4.1 follows from the estimate given in Anikonov and Vishnevskii (1996):

$$\|\lambda(x)\|_{\mathbf{W}_2^{m-2}(D)} \le C'\Bigg(\Big(\sum_{k=1}^{\infty} a_k^2(\,|\lambda_k|^m + 1)\Big)^{1/2} + \Big(\sum_{k=1}^{\infty} b_k^2(\,|\lambda_k|^m + 1)\Big)^{1/2}\Bigg)$$
$$\le C''(\|w_a\|_{\mathbf{W}_2^m(D)} + \|w_b\|_{\mathbf{W}_2^m(D)}).$$

Here C' and C'' are positive constants, as above. For a continuous function $f(t)$ that is negative in some neighborhood of b, an analogous estimate holds and it can be verified using the same argument as above. □

(b) Suppose that **A** is an elliptic operator and its real symbol satisfies the estimates

$$C_2(1 + |\xi|^q) \ge |A_0(\xi)| \ge C_1|\xi|^p \tag{4.4.11}$$

for some positive C_1, C_2; let $q > p > 0$ and suppose that the functions $\widehat{w}_a(\xi)$ and $\widehat{w}_b(\xi)$ are determined from the equations

$$w_a(x) = \int\limits_{\mathbb{R}^n} \widehat{w}_a(\xi) e^{ix\xi} \, d\xi, \qquad w_b(x) = \int\limits_{\mathbb{R}^n} \widehat{w}_b(\xi) e^{ix\xi} \, d\xi,$$

where $\widehat{w}_a(\xi)$ and $\widehat{w}_b(\xi)$ are infinitely differentiable rapidly decreasing functions defined in $\mathbb{R}^n$.

The following notation will be used in the sequel.

$$Z(\alpha, \beta, \xi) = \int\limits_{\alpha}^{\beta} f(p) e^{-pA_0(\xi)} \, dp, \quad [\alpha, \beta] \subseteq [a, b],$$

$$\widehat{\mathcal{V}}_a(\xi) = \widehat{w}_a(\xi) e^{-A_0(\xi)a}, \qquad \widehat{\mathcal{V}}_b(\xi) = \widehat{w}_b(\xi) e^{-A_0(\xi)b},$$

$$\widehat{\mathcal{V}}(\xi, t) = \frac{\widehat{\mathcal{V}}_a(\xi) Z(t, b, \xi) + \widehat{\mathcal{V}}_b(\xi) Z(a, t, \xi)}{Z(a, b, \xi)}. \tag{4.4.12}$$

In the case when $f(t)$ is of constant sign, for the operator A, explicit formulae were obtained in Anikonov (1994) for the solution to the inverse problem (4.4.1), (4.4.2):

$$\mathcal{W}(x, t) = \int\limits_{\mathbb{R}^n} e^{i\xi x} e^{A_0(\xi)t} \, \widehat{\mathcal{V}}(\xi, t) \, d\xi, \tag{4.4.13}$$

$$\Lambda(x) = \int\limits_{\mathbb{R}^n} e^{i\xi x} \frac{\widehat{\mathcal{V}}_b(\xi) - \widehat{\mathcal{V}}_a(\xi)}{Z(a, b, \xi)} \, d\xi. \tag{4.4.14}$$

Let $f(t)$ be a continuous and monotone function on $[a, b]$. We also assume that $f(t)$ changes sign on $[a, b]$: $f(c) = 0$, where $a < c < b$. For definiteness, suppose that $f(t)$ is decreasing. The argument is easily adapted for the case of an increasing function after multiplying $f(t)$ by -1.

Let c_1, c_2 be arbitrary points such that $a < c_1 < c < c_2 < b$. Introduce the notation:

$$f_0 = \frac{1}{b - a} \int\limits_a^b f(t) \, dt, \quad f_1 = \sup_{t \in [a, b]} |f(t)| > 0, \quad f_2 = \inf_{t \in [a, c_1]} |f(t)| > 0,$$

$$f_3 = \inf_{t \in [c, b]} f(t) < 0, \qquad f_4 = \sup_{t \in [c_2, b]} f(t) < 0.$$

In the case $f_0 = 0$, we denote by $\gamma(t)$ the primitive of $f(t)$ that vanishes at the endpoints of $[a, b]$. By the monotonicity of $f(t)$, we have $|\gamma(t)| > 0$ for $a < t < b$.

Theorem 4.4.2. *1) Suppose that the symbol of* $\mathbf{A}$ *satisfies* (4.4.11), $D = \mathbb{R}^n$, *the initial and terminal data* $w_a(x)$ *and* $w_b(x)$ *are rapidly decreasing infinitely differentiable functions, and suppose that* $f(t)$ *is monotone on* $[a, b]$. *Then, if either* $f_0 A_0(\xi) > 0$ *for* $A_0(\xi) \neq 0$ *or* $f_0 = 0$ *and* $p < n$, *then the functions* $\mathcal{W}(x,t)$ *and* $\Lambda(x)$ *which are a solution to the inverse problem* (4.4.1), (4.4.2) *are well defined by* (4.4.13) *and* (4.4.14).

2) If $T_0(x)$ *belongs to the kernel of* $\mathbf{\Lambda}$ *whenever* $f_0 = 0$, *then a solution to* (4.4.1), (4.4.2) *is well defined by the formulae*

$$w(x,t) = \mathcal{W}(x,t) + \gamma(t) T_0(x), \qquad \lambda(x) = \Lambda(x) + T_0(x). \tag{4.4.15}$$

Therefore, whenever $f_0 = 0$, the space of solutions to this problem contains a subspace isomorphic to Ker $\mathbf{A}$.

Proof. Denote

$$Y = \mathrm{e}^{A_0(\xi)t} \left(\widehat{\mathcal{V}}_a(\xi) Z(t, b, \xi) + \widehat{\mathcal{V}}_b(\xi) Z(a, t, \xi) \right).$$

Clearly,

$$|Y| \le \Big(\frac{|\widehat{w}_a(\xi)| \, |\mathrm{e}^{A_0(\xi)(t-a-b)} - \mathrm{e}^{-A_0(\xi)a}|}{|A_0(\xi)|} + \frac{|\widehat{w}_b(\xi)| \, |\mathrm{e}^{-A_0(\xi)b} - \mathrm{e}^{-A_0(\xi)(t-a-b)}|}{|A_0(\xi)|} \Big) f_1.$$

It is noteworthy that, when $\xi = 0$, the denominator on the right-hand side becomes zero, but the assumptions of the theorem imply that, in performing the inverse Fourier transform, this singularity is integrable.

Consider $Z(a, b, \xi) = Z(a, c, \xi) + Z(c, b, \xi)$. The first term of the sum is positive whereas the second is negative. We have

$$\frac{f_1(\mathrm{e}^{-A_0(\xi)c} - \mathrm{e}^{-A_0(\xi)a})}{-A_0(\xi)} > Z(a, c, \xi) > \frac{f_2(\mathrm{e}^{-A_0(\xi)c_1} - \mathrm{e}^{-A_0(\xi)a})}{-A_0(\xi)} > 0,$$

$$0 > \frac{f_4(\mathrm{e}^{-A_0(\xi)b} - \mathrm{e}^{-A_0(\xi)c_2})}{-A_0(\xi)} > Z(c, b, \xi) > \frac{f_3(\mathrm{e}^{-A_0(\xi)b} - \mathrm{e}^{-A_0(\xi)c})}{-A_0(\xi)}$$

and

$$\frac{f_1(\mathrm{e}^{-A_0(\xi)c} - \mathrm{e}^{-A_0(\xi)a}) + f_4(\mathrm{e}^{-A_0(\xi)b} - \mathrm{e}^{-A_0(\xi)c_2})}{-A_0(\xi)} > Z(a, b, \xi)$$
$$> \frac{f_2(\mathrm{e}^{-A_0(\xi)c_1} - \mathrm{e}^{-A_0(\xi)a}) + f_3(\mathrm{e}^{-A_0(\xi)b} - \mathrm{e}^{-A_0(\xi)c})}{-A_0(\xi)}. \tag{4.4.16}$$

1) Let $A_0(\xi) \le G\,|\xi|^p$, where $G < 0$ and $p > 0$. Then, for nonzero $A_0(\xi)$, the left-hand side of the last inequality can be rewritten as

$$\frac{\mathrm{e}^{-A_0(\xi)b}}{-A_0(\xi)}\Big(f_1(\mathrm{e}^{A_0(\xi)(b-c)} - \mathrm{e}^{A_0(\xi)(b-a)}) + f_4(1 - \mathrm{e}^{A_0(\xi)(b-c_2)})\Big).$$

For $|\xi|$ sufficiently large, all the exponents in the above formula become considerably smaller than 1 and, since $f_4 < 0$, the left-hand side becomes negative. Consequently,

$$\begin{aligned}|Z(a,b,\xi)| &> \frac{1}{|A_0(\xi)|}\Big(-f_1(\mathrm{e}^{-A_0(\xi)c} - \mathrm{e}^{-A_0(\xi)a}) - f_4(\mathrm{e}^{-A_0(\xi)b} - \mathrm{e}^{-A_0(\xi)c_2})\Big)\\ &> \frac{1}{|A_0(\xi)|}\Big(\frac{-f_4}{2}\mathrm{e}^{-A_0(\xi)b} - f_1\mathrm{e}^{-A_0(\xi)c}\Big) \qquad (4.4.17)\end{aligned}$$

since $1/2 > \mathrm{e}^{A_0(\xi)(b-c_2)}$ for large $-A_0(\xi)$. In this case,

$$\begin{aligned}\Big|\widehat{\mathcal{V}}(\xi,t)\mathrm{e}^{A_0(\xi)t}\Big| &= \Big|\frac{Y}{Z(a,b,\xi)}\Big|\\ &< \frac{|\widehat{w}_a(\xi)|\,\big|\mathrm{e}^{A_0(\xi)(t-a-b)} - \mathrm{e}^{-A_0(\xi)a}\big| + |\widehat{w}_b(\xi)|\,\big|\mathrm{e}^{-A_0(\xi)b} - \mathrm{e}^{A_0(\xi)(t-a-b)}\big|}{(-f_4/2)\mathrm{e}^{-A_0(\xi)b} - f_1\mathrm{e}^{-A_0(\xi)c}} f_1\\ &\le \frac{2f_1(\,|\widehat{w}_a(\xi)| + |\widehat{w}_b(\xi)|\,)}{(-f_4)\,(1 - (2f_1/(-f_4))\mathrm{e}^{A_0(\xi)(b-c)})} < \frac{4f_1}{-f_4}(\,|\widehat{w}_a(\xi)| + |\widehat{w}_b(\xi)|\,)\end{aligned}$$

for $A_0(\xi)(b-c) < -\ln(4f_1/(-f_4))$.

A similar estimate holds for the function

$$\widehat{\Lambda}(\xi) = \frac{\widehat{w}_b(\xi)\mathrm{e}^{-A_0(\xi)b} - \widehat{w}_a(\xi)\mathrm{e}^{-A_0(\xi)a}}{Z(a,b,\xi)}.$$

For $-A_0(\xi)$ sufficiently large, the denominator of this fraction satisfies (4.4.17) and, in this case,

$$\begin{aligned}\big|\widehat{\Lambda}(\xi)\big| &< \frac{|A_0(\xi)|\,(\,|\widehat{w}_b(\xi)|\,\mathrm{e}^{-A_0(\xi)b} + |\widehat{w}_a(\xi)|\,\mathrm{e}^{-A_0(\xi)a})}{\big|(-f_4/2)\mathrm{e}^{-A_0(\xi)b} - f_1\mathrm{e}^{-A_0(\xi)c_1}\big|}\\ &= \frac{|A_0(\xi)|\,(\,|\widehat{w}_b(\xi)| + |\widehat{w}_a(\xi)|\,\mathrm{e}^{A_0(\xi)(b-a)})}{(-f_4/2)\,\big|1 - (2f_1/(-f_4))\mathrm{e}^{A_0(\xi)(b-c)}\big|} < \frac{4\,|A_0(\xi)|}{-f_4}(\,|\widehat{w}_a(\xi)| + |\widehat{w}_b(\xi)|\,)\end{aligned}$$

if $A_0(\xi)(b-c) < -\ln(4f_1/(-f_4))$.

2) Now suppose that $A_0(\xi) > G\,|\xi|^p$, where $G > 0$ and $p > 0$. For $A_0(\xi)$ sufficiently large, whenever

$$\frac{f_2}{2}\left(1 - e^{A_0(\xi)(a-c_1)}\right) + f_3\left(e^{A_0(\xi)(a-c)} - e^{A_0(\xi)(a-b)}\right) > 0$$

inequalities (4.4.16) take the form

$$\frac{f_1(e^{-A_0(\xi)a} - e^{-A_0(\xi)c})}{A_0(\xi)} > Z(a,b,\xi) > \frac{f_2(e^{-A_0(\xi)a} - e^{-A_0(\xi)c_1})}{2A_0(\xi)} > 0.$$

Therefore,

$$|Z(a,b,\xi)| > \frac{f_2(e^{-A_0(\xi)a} - e^{-A_0(\xi)c_1})}{2A_0(\xi)} > 0,$$

and then

$$|\widehat{\mathcal{V}}(\xi,t)| = \left|\frac{Y}{Z(a,b,\xi)}\right|$$

$$\leq \frac{2f_1\left(|\widehat{w}_a(\xi)|\,\left|e^{A_0(\xi)(t-b)} - 1\right| + |\widehat{w}_b(\xi)|\,\left|e^{A_0(\xi)(a-b)} - e^{A_0(\xi)(t-b)}\right|\right)}{f_2(1 - e^{A_0(\xi)(a-c_1)})}$$

$$\leq \frac{4f_1}{f_2}(\,|\widehat{w}_a(\xi)| + |\widehat{w}_b(\xi)|\,).$$

We hereby established the correctness of (4.4.13) in all cases for both positive and negative $A_0(\xi)$.

In the case $G > 0$, a similar estimate holds for the function $\widehat{\Lambda}(\xi)$. Using the same argument as in the end of the previous section for $|\xi|$ sufficiently large we have

$$|\widehat{\Lambda}(\xi)| < \frac{4\,|A_0(\xi)|}{f_2}(|\widehat{w}_a(\xi)| + |\widehat{w}_b(\xi)|).$$

Since the functions $w_a(x)$ and $w_b(x)$ are rapidly decreasing, the same is true for their Fourier transforms $\widehat{w}_a(\xi)$ and $\widehat{w}_b(\xi)$; therefore, in view of (4.4.11), the function $\widehat{\Lambda}(\xi)$ is also rapidly decreasing, which implies the correctness of the representation (4.4.14).

Let R be a number such that, outside the ball $|\xi| \geq R$, all the above estimates hold and thus ensure the convergence of the integrals (4.4.13) and (4.4.14). Inside this compact ball, their convergence can only be violated provided that $Z(a,b,\xi)$ vanishes.

If $f_0 = 0$, then, as was shown above,

$$f(t) = \frac{d\gamma}{dt}, \qquad \gamma(a) = \gamma(b) = 0$$

and the function $\gamma(t)$ is positive at the interior points of $[a, b]$. In this case, integrating by parts, we have

$$Z(a,b,\xi) = \int_a^b e^{-A_0(\xi)t} f(t)\,dt = A_0(\xi) \int_a^b e^{-A_0(\xi)t}\gamma(t)\,dt. \qquad (4.4.18)$$

This denominator vanishes only when $A_0(\xi) = 0$. For $p < n$, this singularity is integrable.

Now let $f_0 \neq 0$. Denote by $\varphi(t)$ the difference $f(t) - f_0$. Then the integral $\int_a^b e^{-A_0(\xi)t}\varphi(t)\,dt$ has the form (4.4.18). We represent the unknown function $w(x,t)$ as the sum $w(x,t) = w_1(x,t) + w_2(x,t)$ whose terms are solutions to the two inverse problems:

$$\text{I. } \frac{\partial w_1}{\partial t} = Aw_1 + \lambda(x)\varphi(t); \quad w_1(x,a) = w_1(x,b) = w_{a,1}(x);$$

$$\text{II. } \frac{\partial w_2}{\partial t} = Aw_2 + \lambda(x) f_0; \quad \begin{aligned} w_2(x,a) &= w_a(x) - w_{a,1}(x), \\ w_2(x,b) &= w_b(x) - w_{a,1}(x) \end{aligned}$$

with the same function $\lambda(x)$ and still unknown function $w_{a,1}(x)$. For both problems, write down the expression for $\widehat{\lambda}(\xi)$:

$$\text{I. } \widehat{\lambda}(\xi) = \frac{\widehat{w}_{a,1}(\xi)(e^{-A_0(\xi)b} - e^{-A_0(\xi)a})}{\int_a^b e^{-A_0(\xi)t}\varphi(t)\,dt} = \frac{\widehat{w}_{a,1}(\xi)(e^{-A_0(\xi)b} - e^{-A_0(\xi)a})}{A_0(\xi)\int_a^b e^{-A_0(\xi)t}\gamma(t)\,dt};$$

$$\text{II. } \widehat{\lambda}(\xi) = \frac{(\widehat{w}_b(\xi) - \widehat{w}_{a,1}(\xi))e^{-A_0(\xi)b} - (\widehat{w}_a(\xi) - \widehat{w}_{a,1}(\xi))e^{-A_0(\xi)a}}{f_0 \int_a^b e^{-A_0(\xi)t}\,dt}.$$

The denominator in the second formula is nonzero. In the first formula, as $A_0(\xi) \to 0$, the limit of

$$\frac{e^{-A_0(\xi)b} - e^{-A_0(\xi)a}}{A_0(\xi)}$$

is finite. Excluding $\widehat{\lambda}(\xi)$ from these equalities, we obtain the expression from which the unknown function $\widehat{w}_{a,1}(\xi)$ can be found:

$$\widehat{w}_{a,1}(\xi)\frac{e^{-A_0(\xi)b} - e^{-A_0(\xi)a}}{A_0(\xi)}\left(f_0\int_a^b e^{-A_0(\xi)t}\,dt + A_0(\xi)\int_a^b e^{-A_0(\xi)t}\gamma(t)\,dt\right)$$

$$= \left(\widehat{w}_b(\xi)e^{-A_0(\xi)b} - \widehat{w}_a(\xi)e^{-A_0(\xi)a}\right)\int_a^b e^{-A_0(\xi)t}\gamma(t)\,dt.$$

If $f_0 A_0(\xi) > 0$ for $A_0(\xi) \neq 0$, then this equality allows us to find $\widehat{w}_{a,1}(\xi)$, the solutions $w_1(x,t)$ and $w_2(x,t)$ to (I, II), and their sum, which is a solution to the original problem.

Therefore, the proof of the first statement of Theorem 4.4.2 is complete. The validity of the formulae (4.4.15) is verified as in Anikonov (1994) by substituting them into the initial equation (4.4.1) and conditions (4.4.2). □

(c) In this subsection, we consider systems of evolution equations similar to (4.4.1), (4.4.2):

$$\frac{\partial}{\partial t}\mathcal{W}(x,t) = \mathbf{A}\,\mathcal{W}(x,t) + F(t)\Lambda(x) \tag{4.4.19}$$

with initial and terminal conditions

$$\mathcal{W}(x,a) = \mathcal{W}_a(x) \in \mathbb{R}^m, \qquad \mathcal{W}(x,b) = \mathcal{W}_b(x) \in \mathbb{R}^m, \tag{4.4.20}$$

which are known vector functions.

For such an inverse problem, we shall construct and study formal solutions analogous to those obtained in the case of the single equation (4.4.1).

Here we denote by $F(t)$ a known continuous $(m \times m)$-matrix function depending on the real variable $t \in [a,b]$ and $x = (x^1, \dots, x^n) \in D \subseteq \mathbb{R}^n$.

A linear matrix operator $\mathbf{A} = (\mathbf{A}_{l,j})$, $m \geq l, j \geq 1$, acts on the space variables and its components $\mathbf{A}_{l,j}$ have real symbols $a_{l,j}(\xi)$ (see Ladyzhenskaya and Ural'ceva, 1973; Lions and Magenes, 1968), $\mathbf{A}_{l,j}\, e^{i\langle x,\xi\rangle} = a_{l,j}(\xi)e^{i\langle x,\xi\rangle}$, which satisfy the estimates similar to (4.4.11):

$$C_2(1 + |\xi|^q) \geq |a_{l,j}(\xi)| \geq C_1|\xi|^p, \tag{4.4.21}$$

where C_1 and C_2 are positive numbers, $q > p > 0$, $1 \leq l, j \leq m$, and $\xi \in \mathbb{R}^n$.

The unknown functions to be found are the vector functions $\mathcal{W}(x,t)$ and $\Lambda(x) \in \mathbb{R}^m$. As usual, integration and differentiation of matrix and vector functions is performed componentwise.

We seek a solution to the inverse problem (4.4.19), (4.4.20) in the form

$$W(x,t) = \int_{\mathbb{R}^n} \widehat{W}(\xi,t)\mathrm{e}^{\mathrm{i}\langle x,\xi\rangle}\,\mathrm{d}\xi, \qquad \Lambda(x) = \int_{\mathbb{R}^n} \widehat{\Lambda}(\xi)\mathrm{e}^{\mathrm{i}\langle x,\xi\rangle}\,\mathrm{d}\xi, \tag{4.4.22}$$

where the vector functions

$$\begin{gathered} \widehat{W}(\xi,t) = P_a(\xi,t)\widehat{W}_a(\xi) + P_b(\xi,t)\widehat{W}_b(\xi), \\ \widehat{\Lambda}(\xi) = Q_a(\xi)\widehat{W}_a(\xi) + Q_b(\xi)\widehat{W}_b(\xi) \end{gathered} \tag{4.4.23}$$

satisfy the equation

$$\frac{\partial}{\partial t}\widehat{W}(\xi,t) = \mathrm{M}(\xi)\widehat{W}(\xi,t) + F(t)\widehat{\Lambda}(\xi). \tag{4.4.24}$$

Here $P_a(\xi,t)$, $P_b(\xi,t)$, $Q_a(\xi)$, and $Q_a(\xi)$ are $(m\times m)$-matrices that satisfy the boundary-value conditions

$$P_a(\xi,a) = \mathbf{E}, \quad P_a(\xi,b) = \mathbf{0}, \quad P_b(\xi,a) = \mathbf{0}, \quad P_b(\xi,b) = \mathbf{E}, \tag{4.4.25}$$

where $\mathbf{E}$ and $\mathbf{0}$ denote the unit and zero $(m \times m)$-matrices, and the matrix $\mathrm{M}(\xi) = (a_{l,j}(\xi))$ consists of the symbols of operators $\mathbf{A}_{l,j}$.

Substituting such functions $\widehat{W}(\xi,t)$ and $\widehat{\Lambda}(\xi)$ into (4.4.24), we require that the formulae (4.4.23) determine a solution to this equation for arbitrary initial and terminal conditions $\widehat{W}_a(\xi)$ and $\widehat{W}_a(\xi)$. In such general case, we obtain the following matrix differential equations:

$$\frac{\partial P_a}{\partial t} = \mathrm{M}(\xi)P_a(\xi,t) + F(t)Q_a(\xi), \tag{4.4.26}$$

$$\frac{\partial P_b}{\partial t} = \mathrm{M}(\xi)P_b(\xi,t) + F(t)Q_b(\xi), \tag{4.4.27}$$

whose solutions have the following form (see Gantmaher, 1966):

$$P_a(\xi,t) = -\exp\Big(\mathrm{M}(\xi)(t-a)\Big)\int_t^b \exp\Big(\mathrm{M}(\xi)(a-\tau)\Big)F(\tau)Q_a(\xi)\,\mathrm{d}\tau,$$

$$P_b(\xi,t) = \exp\Big(\mathrm{M}(\xi)(t-b)\Big)\int_a^t \exp\Big(\mathrm{M}(\xi)(b-\tau)\Big)F(\tau)Q_b(\xi)\,\mathrm{d}\tau.$$

Here the matrices $Q_a(\xi)$ and $Q_b(\xi)$ are determined from (4.4.25):

$$-\mathbf{E} = \Big(\int_a^b \exp\big(\mathrm{M}(\xi)(a-\tau)\big)F(\tau)\,\mathrm{d}\tau\Big)Q_a(\xi), \tag{4.4.28}$$

$$\mathbf{E} = \Big(\int_a^b \exp\big(\mathrm{M}(\xi)(b-\tau)\big)F(\tau)\,\mathrm{d}\tau\Big)Q_b(\xi). \tag{4.4.29}$$

Introduce the notation:

$$\varphi_a(\xi,\tau) = \exp\big(\mathrm{M}(\xi)(a-\tau)\big)F(\tau), \qquad \varphi_b(\xi,\tau) = \exp\big(\mathrm{M}(\xi)(b-\tau)\big)F(\tau)$$

$$\Phi_a(\xi) = \int_a^b \varphi_a(\xi,\tau)\,\mathrm{d}\tau, \qquad \Phi_b(\xi) = \int_a^b \varphi_b(\xi,\tau)\,\mathrm{d}\tau.$$

Then equations (4.4.28) and (4.4.29) can be rewritten as

$$-\mathbf{E} = \Phi_a(\xi)Q_a(\xi), \qquad \mathbf{E} = \Phi_b(\xi)Q_b(\xi)$$

and thus, in order to find $Q_a(\xi)$ and $Q_b(\xi)$, which are involved in the explicit expression for the needed vector functions $\widehat{\mathcal{W}}(\xi,t)$ and $\widehat{\Lambda}(\xi)$, we have to invert the matrices $\Phi_a(\xi)$ and $\Phi_b(\xi)$ for all $\xi \in \mathbb{R}^n$ in such a way that the inverse Fourier transform would give regular vector functions $\mathcal{W}(x,t)$ and $\Lambda(x)$.

We give a sufficient condition for such invertibility. Suppose that the factors of the matrices $\varphi_a(\xi,t)$ and $\varphi_b(\xi,t)$, namely,

$$F(\tau), \quad \exp\big(\mathrm{M}(\xi)(a-\tau)\big), \quad \exp\big(\mathrm{M}(\xi)(b-\tau)\big), \tag{4.4.30}$$

are such that the inequality

$$\langle By, y\rangle > \rho\,|y|\,|By| \tag{4.4.31}$$

holds for all nonzero $y \in \mathbb{R}^m$ and all $\tau \in [a,b]$. Here B is any of the matrices listed in (4.4.30) and ρ is a number in the interval $(\sqrt{2}/2, 1)$.

A geometric interpretation of this condition is that the direction of nonzero vectors changes by less than $\pi/4$ under multiplication by such a matrix and therefore multiplication by $\varphi_a(\xi,\tau)$ and $\varphi_a(\xi,\tau)$ changes the direction of a vector x by an angle $\alpha(x) < \alpha_0 = \arccos(2\rho^2 - 1) < \pi/2$. This implies the invertibility of such matrices.

Theorem 4.4.3. *Suppose that the initial and terminal data* (4.4.20) *for system* (4.4.19) *are rapidly decreasing infinitely differentiable functions,* $D = \mathbb{R}^n$ *and, for all* $\xi \in \mathbb{R}^n$, *conditions* (4.4.21) *and* (4.4.31) *hold. Suppose that the matrix* $\mathrm{M}(\xi)$ *is symmetric and its eigenvalues are of the same sign. Then a solution* $W(x,t)$, $\Lambda(x)$ *to the inverse problem* (4.4.19), (4.4.20) *is well defined by formulae* (4.4.22).

Proof. First of all, we observe that the norm $\|\mathrm{M}(\xi)\|$ of the matrix $\mathrm{M}(\xi)$ and its eigenvalues $\mu_1(\xi), \dots, \mu_m(\xi)$ satisfy estimates (4.4.21) too, which readily follows if we apply an orthogonal transformation to the basis of eigenvectors of $\mathrm{M}(\xi)$. Derive a lower bound for the norms of $\Phi_a(\xi)$ and $\Phi_a(\xi)$. Given a nonsingular matrix B, denote by $\delta(B)$ the minimal value of $|Bx|$ over all unit vectors $x \in S^{m-1} \subset \mathbb{R}^m$. Obviously,

$$\delta(\varphi_a(\xi,\tau)) = \|\varphi_a^{-1}(\xi,\tau)\|^{-1} \geq \|F^{-1}(\tau)\|^{-1} \|\exp(\mathrm{M}(\xi)(\tau - a))\|^{-1}.$$

Let F_0 be the maximal value of $\|F^{-1}(\tau)\|$ on $[a,b]$. Then

$$\|\varphi_a^{-1}(\xi,\tau)\|^{-1} \geq (F_0)^{-1} \|\exp(\mathrm{M}(\xi)(\tau - a))\|^{-1}$$

and since

$$\exp(\|\mathrm{M}(\xi)\|(\tau - a)) \geq \|\exp(\mathrm{M}(\xi)(\tau - a))\| \geq \exp(-\|\mathrm{M}(\xi)\|(\tau - a))$$

(see, for example, Godunov, 1994), after integrating over $[a,b]$ an inequality equivalent to $\cos\alpha(x) \geq 2\rho^2 - 1$, for unit vectors x we obtain

$$\left| \int_a^b \exp(\mathrm{M}(\xi)(a-\tau)) F(\tau) x \, \mathrm{d}\tau \right| \geq \left\langle \int_a^b \exp(\mathrm{M}(\xi)(a-\tau)) F(\tau) x \, \mathrm{d}\tau,\, x \right\rangle$$

$$\geq (2\rho^2 - 1) \int_a^b |\exp(\mathrm{M}(\xi)(a-\tau)) F(\tau) x| \, \mathrm{d}\tau$$

$$\geq \frac{2\rho^2 - 1}{F_0} \int_a^b \exp(\|\mathrm{M}(\xi)\|(a-\tau)) \, \mathrm{d}\tau = \frac{2\rho^2 - 1}{F_0 \|\mathrm{M}(\xi)\|} (1 - \exp(\|\mathrm{M}(\xi)\|(a-b))).$$

Similarly, it can be shown that the following inequality holds for unit vectors $x \in S^{m-1}$:

$$\left| \int_a^b \exp(\mathrm{M}(\xi)(b-\tau)) F(\tau) x \, \mathrm{d}\tau \right| \geq \frac{2\rho^2 - 1}{F_0 \|\mathrm{M}(\xi)\|} \Big(1 - \exp(\|\mathrm{M}(\xi)\|(a-b))\Big).$$

These estimates have an obvious geometric interpretation. The integration of a vector function whose range is included in a convex cone with vertex in the origin gives a nonzero result.

Denote by $C(\xi)$ the right-hand side of the last two inequalities. Apparently, it has finite limit $\dfrac{2\rho^2-1}{F_0(b-a)}$ as $\|\,\mathrm{M}(\xi)\| \to 0$.

Thus, the norms of the matrices $-Q_a(\xi)$ and $Q_b(\xi)$ inverse to the matrices $\Phi_a(\xi)$ and $\Phi_b(\xi)$ do not exceed

$$C(\xi)^{-1} = \frac{F_0}{2\rho^2-1}\|\mathrm{M}(\xi)\|\Big(1-\exp\left(\|\mathrm{M}(\xi)\|(a-b)\right)\Big)^{-1},$$

which satisfies (4.4.21) as was shown above.

Therefore, the vector function $\widehat{\Lambda}(\xi) = Q_a(\xi)\widehat{W}_a(\xi) + Q_b(\xi)\widehat{W}_b(\xi)$ is well defined and, by (4.4.21), it is rapidly decreasing in ξ. Note that, since multiplication by $\Phi_a(\xi)$ and $\Phi_b(\xi)$ takes the vectors from the unit ball $D(1) \subset \mathbb{R}^m$ to ellipsoids that contain the ball $D(C(\xi))$ of radius $C(\xi)$, the determinants of both of these matrices are not less than $C(\xi)^m$, which is the quotient of the volumes of $D(C(\xi))$ and $D(1)$.

Suppose that the eigenvalues of $\mathrm{M}(\xi)$ are positive for all $\xi \in \mathbb{R}^n$. Fixing an arbitrary ξ, find the diagonal form of $\mathrm{M}(\xi)$ and rewrite the Fourier transform of the solution to the matrix equation (4.4.19) as follows:

$$\begin{aligned}
\widehat{W}(\xi,t) &= \exp\left(\mathrm{M}(\xi)(t-a)\right)\left[-\int_t^b \exp\left(\mathrm{M}(\xi)(a-\tau)\right)F(\tau)\,\mathrm{d}\tau\right]Q_a(\xi)\widehat{W}_a(\xi) \\
&\quad + \exp\left(\mathrm{M}(\xi)(t-b)\right)\left[\int_a^t \exp\left(\mathrm{M}(\xi)(b-\tau)\right)F(\tau)\,\mathrm{d}\tau\right]Q_b(\xi)\widehat{W}_b(\xi) \\
&= \exp\left(\mathrm{M}(\xi)(t-b)\right)\left[\int_a^b - \int_t^b\right]\Big(\exp\left(\mathrm{M}(\xi)(b-\tau)\right)F(\tau)\,\mathrm{d}\tau\Big)Q_b(\xi)\widehat{W}_b(\xi) \\
&\quad -\left[\int_t^b \exp\left(\mathrm{M}(\xi)(t-\tau)\right)F(\tau)\,\mathrm{d}\tau\right]Q_a(\xi)\widehat{W}_a(\xi) \\
&= \exp\left(\mathrm{M}(\xi)(t-b)\right)\widehat{W}_b(\xi) - \left[\int_t^b \exp\left(\mathrm{M}(\xi)(t-\tau)\right)F(\tau)\,\mathrm{d}\tau\right]\widehat{\Lambda}(\xi).
\end{aligned}$$

All the exponents in the last expression are diagonal matrices whose elements do not exceed 1; therefore, the modulus of the subtrahend in the last formula is less than

$$|\widehat{\Lambda}(\xi)|F_0 \max_{j=1,\dots,m} \left[\frac{1}{\mu_j(\xi)}\Big(1 - \mathrm{e}^{\mu_j(\xi)(t-b)}\Big)\right],$$

which is a rapidly decreasing function in ξ.

In the case when the eigenvalues of $\mathrm{M}(\xi)$ are negative for all $\xi \in \mathbb{R}^n$, the same type of argument with negative exponents of a diagonal matrix can be used for the expression

$$\widehat{W}(\xi,t) = \left[\int_a^t \exp\big(\mathrm{M}(\xi)(t-\tau)\big)F(\tau)\,\mathrm{d}\tau\right] Q_b(\xi)\widehat{W}_b(\xi)$$

$$- \exp\big(\mathrm{M}(\xi)(t-a)\big)\left[\int_a^b - \int_a^t\right]\Big(\exp\big(\mathrm{M}(\xi)(a-\tau)\big)F(\tau)\,\mathrm{d}\tau\Big) Q_a(\xi)\widehat{W}_a(\xi)$$

$$= \exp\big(\mathrm{M}(\xi)(t-a)\big)\widehat{W}_a(\xi) + \left[\int_a^t \exp\big(\mathrm{M}(\xi)(t-\tau)\big)F(\tau)\,\mathrm{d}\tau\right]\widehat{\Lambda}(\xi).$$

Therefore, the vector function $\widehat{W}(\xi,t)$ is also rapidly decreasing in ξ and thus a solution to the original inverse problem is well defined by (4.4.22). This proves Theorem 4.4.3. □

Theorem 4.4.4. *Let the initial and terminal data* (4.4.20) *for system* (4.4.19) *belong to the class of entire functions* $\{\varphi(z);\ z = x + \mathrm{i}y\}$ *with components satisfying the inequality*

$$|\varphi(x+\mathrm{i}y)| \le C_\varepsilon \mathrm{e}^{(N+\varepsilon)|y|}(1+|x|)^s,$$

where $C_\varepsilon > 0$, $N > 0$, $s \ge 0$, $\varepsilon > 0$. *Suppose that* $D \subset \mathbb{R}^n$ *and, for all* $\xi \in \mathbb{R}^n$ *such that* $|\xi| < N + \varepsilon_0$ *and* $\varepsilon_0 > 0$, *conditions* (4.4.31) *hold and* $\mathrm{M}(\xi)$ *is symmetric with eigenvalues of the same sign. Then an entire (in* x*) solution* $W(x,t)$, $\Lambda(x)$ *to the inverse problem* (4.4.19), (4.4.20) *is well defined by formulae* (4.4.22).

Proof. The statement of the theorem follows from the invertibility of $\Phi_a(\xi)$ and $\Phi_b(\xi)$ inside the ball $D(N+\varepsilon_0) \subset \mathbb{R}^n$, which, according to the theorem of Paley – Wiener – Schwartz, contains the supports of the vector functions $\widehat{W}_a(\xi)$ and $\widehat{W}_b(\xi)$. Therefore, the functions integrated in (4.4.22) have compact supports as in the case of the single equation (4.4.1). Thus, the required vector functions are entire in x. Direct calculation shows that they form a solution to the inverse problem (4.4.19), (4.4.20). □

In the theory of nonlinear dynamic systems, these configurations of the eigenvalues of the matrix $M(\xi)$ correspond to the Poincare domain (see Arnol'd, 1988). Here the trajectories of the systems have "regular" behaviour in contrast with the Siegel domain. In this case the convex hulls of the eigenvalues contain the zero point of the complex plane.

Note that the invertibility conditions for $\Phi_a(\xi)$ and $\Phi_b(\xi)$ that we have just considered do not comprise many of those cases in which systems of the form (4.4.19) arise. For instance, reducing the evolution equation of the second order, $w_{tt} + \mathbf{A}\, w = \lambda_1(x) f_1(t) + \lambda_2(x) f_2(t)$ (see Anikonov, 1995), to an equation of the form (4.4.19), we obtain an expression for the explicit solution to the inverse problem involving the matrices

$$M(\xi) = \begin{pmatrix} 0 & \sqrt{A(\xi)} \\ -\sqrt{A(\xi)} & 0 \end{pmatrix}, \qquad F(t) = \begin{pmatrix} 0 & 0 \\ f_1(x) & f_2(x) \end{pmatrix}. \tag{4.4.32}$$

Here $A(\xi)$ is the symbol of the operator $\mathbf{A}$. In this case, $\Phi_a(\xi)$ is the inverse to the matrix

$$\begin{pmatrix} \int_a^b f_1(t) \cdot \sin(\sqrt{A(\xi)}(a-t))\, dt & \int_a^b f_2(t) \cdot \sin(\sqrt{A(\xi)}(a-t))\, dt \\ \int_a^b f_1(t) \cdot \cos(\sqrt{A(\xi)}(a-t))\, dt & \int_a^b f_2(t) \cdot \cos(\sqrt{A(\xi)}(a-t))\, dt \end{pmatrix}. \tag{4.4.33}$$

The inverse of $\Phi_b(\xi)$ has a similar expression.

Denote by $\Pi(f_1, f_2)$ the two-dimensional plane in $L_2[a,b]$ spanned by the vectors f_1 and f_2.

Lemma 4.4.1. *For every pair of functions $f_1, f_2 \in L_2[a,b]$, the matrix (4.4.33) is singular for countably many values of $\sqrt{A(\xi)}$.*

Note that the determinant of this matrix equals up to the sign, the product of the area of the parallelogram spanned by f_1 and f_2 and the area of the parallelogram spanned by the projections of $\sin(\sqrt{A(\xi)}\,(a-t))$ and $\cos(\sqrt{A(\xi)}\,(a-t))$ on the plane $\Pi(f_1, f_2)$. The geometric meaning of the statement of the lemma is that, for all such functions f_1 and f_2, the orthogonal projection of the two-dimensional plane $\Pi(\xi)$ spanned by the vectors $\sin(\sqrt{A(\xi)}\,(a-t))$ and $\cos(\sqrt{A(\xi)}\,(a-t))$ of the Hilbert space onto the plane $\Pi(f_1, f_2)$ degenerates for countably many values of $\sqrt{A(\xi)}$. Therefore, Theorem 4.4.3 does not hold in the case of skew-symmetric matrices.

Proof. On the standard two-dimensional plane with polar coordinate system $(\alpha, \sqrt{A(\xi)}\,)$, we consider the ring

$$R_{1,2} = \left\{0 \leq \alpha < 2\pi;\quad \frac{2\pi l_1}{b-a} = \beta_1 \leq \sqrt{A(\xi)} \leq \frac{2\pi l_2}{b-a} = \beta_2\right\},$$

where $l_2 > l_1$ are natural numbers and α is the angular coordinate.

Suppose that there exist $f_1, f_2 \in L_2[a,b]$ such that, for all $\sqrt{A(\xi)} \in [\beta_1, \beta_2]$, the plane $\Pi(\xi)$ is biuniquely projected onto $\Pi(f_1, f_2)$. This implies that, for every $\alpha \in [0, 2\pi]$, the integrals

$$I_j\left(\alpha, \sqrt{A(\xi)}\right) = \int_a^b \sin\left(\sqrt{A(\xi)}\,t + \alpha\right) f_j(t)\, \mathrm{d}t, \quad j = 1,2 \qquad (4.4.34)$$

do not vanish simultaneously and that the image of the map

$$I : R_{1,2} \longrightarrow \mathbb{R}^2, \qquad I\left(\alpha, \sqrt{A(\xi)}\right) = (I_1(\xi,\alpha), I_2(\xi,\alpha)) \qquad (4.4.35)$$

does not contain the origin $0 \in \mathbb{R}^2$. It is easy to see that the image of the circle $\sqrt{A(\xi)} = \beta_1$ under I is a closed curve whose index with respect to the origin is $l_1 k_1$, where k_1 is an integer. The corresponding image of the circle $\sqrt{A(\xi)} = \beta_2$ equals $l_2 k_2$. If l_2 has a prime divisor that does not divide $l_1 k_1$, then the boundary components of the ring $R_{1,2}$ have images whose indices with respect to the origin in $\mathbb{R}^2$ are distinct; therefore, for some $\sqrt{A(\xi)} \in [\beta_1, \beta_2]$, there exists a vector $\sin(\sqrt{A(\xi)}\,t + \alpha) \in \Pi(\xi)$ whose orthogonal projection onto the plane $\Pi(f_1, f_2)$ is zero.

In order to prove that the sequence of these values of $\sqrt{A(\xi)}$ is countable, we can similarly construct a sequence of expanding concentric rings $R_{2,3}, R_{3,4}, \ldots$ covering $0 \in \mathbb{R}^2$ under the maps I that are defined by formulae analogous to (4.4.34) and (4.4.35). □

On the other hand, suppose that $M(\xi)$ is skew-symmetric as above and that $F(t)$ has the form

$$F(t) = f(t) \cdot \begin{pmatrix} \cos\alpha(t) & \sin\alpha(t) \\ -\sin\alpha(t) & \cos\alpha(t) \end{pmatrix}, \qquad (4.4.36)$$

where $f(t)$ is a smooth strictly monotone positive function and $\alpha(t)$ is a smooth decreasing function such that, for all $t \in [a, b]$,

$$\frac{\mathrm{d}}{\mathrm{d}t}\left(\frac{f(t)}{|\alpha'(t)|}\right) > 0. \tag{4.4.37}$$

Then $\Phi_a(\xi)$ and $\Phi_b(\xi)$ are invertible in view of the following lemma.

Lemma 4.4.2. *For all $\omega \geq 0$ and $f(t)$ defined above, the integrals*

$$\int_a^b f(t) \cos(\omega(a-t))\, \mathrm{d}t, \qquad \int_a^b f(t) \sin(\omega(a-t))\, \mathrm{d}t$$

do not vanish simultaneously.

The geometric meaning of this fact is that the integral of a vector function that draws a monotonically unfolding (or folding) spiral on an interval is nonzero. The conditions on $f(t)$ and $\alpha(t)$ guarantee the monotonicity of such a spiral.

Proof. The proof of the lemma is easily derived from the following statement:

The Fourier sine transform of a function $f(t)$ that decreases on $(0, +\infty)$ and such that $\lim_{t\to\infty} f(t) = 0$ is a positive function (see Fichtenholz, 1968, V. 3, Chapter XIX, Section 692, Item 14). □

The properties of the Fourier transform imply that the norms of the matrices $\Phi_a(\xi)$ and $\Phi_b(\xi)$ tend to zero as $|\xi| \to \infty$. The rate of the decrease depends on the analytical properties of $f(t)$ and $\alpha(t)$, but, in any case, we have the following analogue of Theorem 4.4.4:

Theorem 4.4.5. *Let the initial and terminal conditions* (4.4.20) *for the system* (4.4.19) *belong to the class of entire matrix functions $\{\varphi(z);\ z = x + \mathrm{i}y\}$ such that*

$$|\varphi(x + \mathrm{i}y)| \leq C_\varepsilon \mathrm{e}^{(N+\varepsilon)|y|}(1 + |x|)^s,$$

where $C_\varepsilon > 0$, $N > 0$, $s \geq 0$, and $\varepsilon > 0$. Suppose that $D \subset \mathbb{R}^n$, the matrices $M(\xi)$ and $F(t)$ are defined by (4.4.32) *and* (4.4.36), *respectively, for all $\xi \in \mathbb{R}^n$ such that $|\xi| < N + \varepsilon_0$, where $\varepsilon_0 > 0$ and, for $t \in [a, b]$, the smooth and strictly monotone positive function $f(t)$ and the smooth decreasing* *function* $\alpha(t)$ *satisfy* (4.4.37). *Then an entire (in* x*) solution* $W(x,t)$, $\Lambda(x)$ *to the inverse problem* (4.4.19), (4.4.20) *is well defined by formulae* (4.4.22).

In a similar way, the problem (4.4.19), (4.4.20) can be studied in the case of matrix functions $\mathcal{W}(x,t)$ and $\Lambda(x)$ (see Ayupova and Golubyatnikov, 1997). In particular, analogues of Theorem 4.4.5 hold for the matrix evolution equation

$$\frac{\partial}{\partial t}\mathcal{W}(x,t) = A\mathcal{W} - \mathcal{W}A + F(t)\Lambda(x) - \Lambda(x)F(t)$$

in the case when the matrix of symbols of A is skew-symmetric and some other restrictions are imposed on the initial and terminal data $\mathcal{W}(x,a)$ and $\mathcal{W}(x,b)$.

Bibliography

Aben, H. K. (1979). *Integrated Photoelasticity.* McGraw-Hill, New York.

Adams, J. F. (1962). Vector fields on spheres. *Ann. of Math.*, 75, 603 – 632.

Aizenberg, L. A., Yuzhakov, A. P. (1983). *Integral Representations and Residues in Multidimensional Complex Analysis.* Transl. Math. Monographs, 58, AMS, Providence.

Aleksandrov, A. D. (1937). On the theory of mixed volumes for convex bodies. Pt II. New inequalities between mixed volumes and their applications. *Mat. Sbornik (N.S.)*, 2 (44), 1205–1238 (in Russian).

Anikonov, Yu. E. (1969). A uniqueness theorem for convex surfaces. *Math. Notes*, 6, 528–529.

Anikonov, Yu. E. and Stepanov, V. N. (1981). Uniqueness and stability of the solution of a problem of geometry in the large. *Math. USSR-Sb.*, 44, 483–490 (in Russian).

Anikonov, Yu. E. (1994). Formulas in a multidimensional inverse problem for an evolution equation. *Mat. Dokl.*, 49, 63–64 (in Russian).

Anikonov, Yu. E. (1995a). *Multidimensional Inverse and Ill-Posed Problems for Differential Equations.* VSP, Utrecht.

Anikonov, Yu. E. (1995b). Analytical representation of solutions to multidimensional inverse problems for evolution equations. *J. Inv. Ill-Posed Problems*, 3, 259–267.

Anikonov, Yu. E. and Vishnevskii, M. P. (1996). Formulas in an inverse problem for an evolution equation. *Siberian Math. J.*, 37, 847–859.

Antsiferov, V. V., Smirnov, G. I., Ustyugov, Yu. A., and Chesnokov, Yu. S. (1997). *Principles of High-Informative Location.* Siberian State University if Railway Communications, Novosibirsk (in Russian).

Arnol'd, V. I. (1978). *Mathematical Methods of Classical Mechanics.* Springer-Verlag, New York - Heidelberg - Berlin.

Arnol'd, V. I. (1988). *Geometrical Methods in the Theory of Ordinary Differential Equations.* Grundlehren der Mathematischen Wissenschaften. Springer-Verlag, New York - Heidelberg - Berlin.

Arnol'd, V. I., Gusein-Zade, S. M., and Varchenko, A. N. (1985). *Singularities of Differentiable Maps.* Monographs in mathematics, 82. Birkhäuser Boston, Inc., Boston.

Ayupova, N. B. and Golubyatnikov, V. P. (1990). Algorithms of solutions of multidimensional inverse problems and complexes of lines and planes. In: *Methods for Solutions of Inverse Problems.* Institute of Mathematics, Novosibirsk, 36–44 (in Russian).

Ayupova, N. B. and Golubyatnikov, V. P. (1997). Inverse problems for evolution equations and matrix Fourier transform. *J. Inv. Ill-Posed Problems,* 5, 401–409.

Ayupova, N. B. and Golubyatnikov, V. P. (1998). On formal solutions to multidimensional evolution equations. *Siberian Adv. Math.*, 8, 21–40.

Ball, K. M. (1991). Shadows of convex bodies. *Trans. Amer. Math. Soc.*, 327, 891–901.

Blagoveshchenskii, A. S. (1986). On reconstruction of a function from known integrals of it, taken along linear manifolds. *Mat. Zametki,* 39, 841–849 (in Russian).

Blaschke, W. (1949). *Kreis und Kugel.* Chelsea, New York.

Bonnesen, T. and Fenchel, W. (1987). *Theory of Convex Bodies.* BSC Associates, Moscow - Idaho.

Bott, R. (1954). Nondegenerate critical manifolds. *Annals of Math.*, 60 (2), 248–261.

Campi, S. (1986). Reconstructing a convex surface from certain inequalities. *Boll. Unione Math. Italiana,* 5B, 945–959.

Chakerian, G. D. (1970). Is a body spherical if all its projections have the same I.Q.? *Amer. Math. Monthly*, 77, 989–992.

Chakerian, G. D. and Groemer, H. (1983). Convex bodies of constant width. In: *Convexity and Its Applications* (Eds. P. M. Gruber and J. M. Wills). Birkhäuser, Basel, 49–96.

Chakerian, G. D. and Lutwak, E. (1992). On the Petty-Schneider theorem. *Contemporary Math.*, 140, 31–37.

Červeny, V., Molotkov, I. A., and Pšenčik, I. (1977). *Ray Method in Seismology.* Univ. Karlova, Praha.

Egglestone, H. G. (1958). *Convexity.* Cambridge University Press, Cambridge.

Fichtenholz, G. M. (1968). *Differential- und Integralrechnung. Vol. 1–3.* VEB Deutscher Verlag der Wissenschaften, Berlin.

Finch, D. V. (1985). Cone beam reconstruction with source on a curve. *SIAM Journal Appl. Math.*, 45, 665–671.

Fomenko, A. T. (1995). *Symplectic Geometry, Methods and Applications.* Advanced study in contemporary mathematics, 5. Gordon and Breach Publishers, Amsterdam.

Fomenko, A. T. and Mishchenko, A. S. (1981). Integrating of the Hamiltonian systems with noncommuting symmetries. In: *Proc. of the Seminar on Vector and Tensor Analysis. Vol. XX.* Moscow University, 5–54 (in Russian).

Gantmaher, F. R. (1966). *Matrizentheorie.* VEB Deutscher Verlag der Wissenschaften, Berlin.

Gardner, R. J. and McMullen, P. (1980). On Hammer's X-ray problem. *Journal London Math. Society*, 2 (21), 171–175.

Gardner, R. J. (1992). X-rays of polygons. *Discrete Comput. Geometry*, 7, 281–293.

Gardner, R. J. and Volčič, A. (1994a). Convex bodies with similar projections, *Proc. Amer. Math. Society*, 121, 563–568.

Gardner, R. J. and Volčič, A. (1994b). Tomography of convex and star bodies. *Advances in Math.*, 108, 367–399.

Gardner, R.J. (1995). *Geometric Tomography.* Cambridge University Press, Cambridge.

Gardner, R. J., Koldobsky, A., and Schlumprecht, T. (1999). An analytic solution to the Busemann-Petty problem. *Annals of Mathematics*, 149, 691–703.

Gel'fand, I. M., Graev, M. I., and Shapiro, Z. Ya. (1967). Integral geometry on k-dimensional planes. *Functional Anal. Appl.*, 1, 15–21.

Gel'fand, I. M., Gindikin, S. G., and Graev, M. I. (1980). Integral geometry in the affine and projective spaces. *Modern Problems of Mathematics*, 10, 53–226.

Gel'fand, I. M. and Graev, M. I. (1968). Complexes of straight lines in the space $\mathbb{C}^n$. *Functional Anal. Appl.*, 2, 39–52.

Godunov, S. K. (1997). *Ordinary Differential Equations with Constant Coefficients, Boundary Value Problem. Vol. 1.* Transl. Math. Monographs, 169, AMS, Providence.

Golubyatnikov, V. P. (1978). A condition for uniqueness of shortest paths. In: *Inverse Problems for Differential Equations of Mathematical Physics.* Computing Center, Novosibirsk, 51–54 (in Russian).

Golubyatnikov, V. P. (1982a). On the tomography of polyhedra. In: *Questions of Well-Posedness in Inverse Problems of Mathematical Physics.* Computing Center, Novosibirsk, 75–76 (in Russian).

Golubyatnikov, V. P. (1982b). On recovering of the shape of a body from its projections. *Soviet Math. Dokl.*, 25, 62–63.

Golubyatnikov, V. P. (1986). Some cohomotopy properties of Thom spaces. *Sibirsk. Mat. Zh.*, 27 (2), 202–205 (in Russian).

Golubyatnikov, V. P. (1988). Unique determination of visible bodies from their projections. *Siberian Math. J.*, 29, 761–764.

Golubyatnikov, V. P. (1990). *Some Inverse Problem in Geometry.* Quaderno n.29/1990, Università degli studi di Milano.

Golubyatnikov, V. P. (1991). On unique recoverability of convex and visible compacta from their projections I. *Math. USSR-Sb.*, 73, 1–10.

Golubyatnikov, V. P. (1992a). Stability problems in certain inverse problems of reconstruction of convex compact sets from their projections. *Siberian Math. J.*, 33, 409–414.

Golubyatnikov, V. P. (1992b). Questions of stability in recovering certain compact sets from their projections. *Soviet Math. Dokl.*, 45, 12–14.

Golubyatnikov, V. P. (1995a). On unique recoverability of convex and visible compacta from their projections II. *Siberian Math. J.*, 36 (2), 265–269.

Golubyatnikov, V. P. (1995b). On uniqueness of reconstruction of the form of convex and visible bodies from their projections. *Amer. Math. Soc. Transl.*, 2 (163), 35–45.

Golubyatnikov, V. P. (1995c) Inverse problem for the Hamilton-Jacobi equation. *J. Inv. Ill-Posed Problems*, 3, 407–410.

Golubyatnikov, V. P. (1997). Inverse problem for the Hamilton-Jacobi equation on a closed manifold. *Siberian Math. J.*, 38, 235–238.

Golubyatnikov, V. P., Pekmen, U., Karaca, I., Ozyilmaz, E., and Tantay, B. (1999). On reconstruction of surfaces from their apparent contours and the stationary phase observation. In: *Proc. Intern. Conf. on Shape Modelling and Applications. Aizu-Wakamatsu, March 1999.* IEEE Computer Society Press, 116–120.

Golubyatnikov, V. P. (1999). On unique recoverability of convex compacta from their projections. The case of complex spaces. *Siberian Math. J.*, 40 (4), 678–681.

Gol'din, S. V. (1997) To the theory of the ray seismic tomography. Parts 1; 2. *Russian Geology and Geophysics*, 37 (5), 1–17; 37 (9), 11–22.

Groemer, H. (1987). Stability theorems for projections of convex sets. *Israel Journal of Math.*, 60, 177–190.

Groemer, H. (1994). Stability results for convex bodies and related spherical integral transforms. *Advances in Math.*, 109, 45–74.

Guillemin, V. and Sternberg, S. (1982). Convexity properties of the moment mappings. *Inventions Mathematicae* 67, 491–513.

Guillemin, V. and Sternberg, S. (1984). Convexity properties of the moment mappings. II. *Inventions Mathematicae*, 67, 533–546.

Hadwiger, H. (1963). Seitenrisse konvexer Körper und Homothetie. *Elem. Math.*, 18, 97–98.

Haefliger, A. (1960). Quelques remarques sur les applications différentiables d'une surface dans le plan. *Ann. Inst. Fourier*, 10, 47–60.

Helgason, S. (1980). *The Radon Transform.* Birkhäuser, Basel – Stuttgart.

Helgason, S. (1984). *Groups and Geometric Analysis. Integral Geometry, Invariant Differential Operators and Spherical Functions.* Academic Press, Orlando.

Kireitov, V. R. (1983). *Inverse Problems of the Photometry.* Computing Center, Novosibirsk (in Russian).

Kirillov, A. A. (1961). On one problem of I. M. Gel'fand. *Soviet Math. Dokl.*, 137, 267–277.

Kuz'minykh, A. V. (1973). Recovery of a convex body from the set of its projections. *Siberian Math. J.*, 25, 284–288.

Ladyzhenskaya, O. A. and Ural'ceva, N. N. (1968). *Linear and Quasilinear Elliptic Equations.* Mathematics in science and engineering, 46. Academic Press, New York – London.

Lighthill, M. I. and Whitham, G. B. (1955). On kinematic waves. *Proc. of Royal Society*, A229, 281–293.

Lions, J.-L. and Magenes, E. (1968). *Problèmes aux Limites non Homogènes et Applications. Vol. 1.* Dunod, Paris.

Minkowsky, H. (1911). Über die Körper konstanter Breite. In: *Gesammelten Werke. Vol. 2.* Teubner, Leipzig – Berlin, 277–279.

Montejano, L. (1991a). Convex bodies with homothetic sections. *Bull. London Math. Society*, 23, 381–386.

Montejano, L. (1991b). A characterization of the Euclidean ball in terms of concurrent sections of constant width. *Geometriae Dedicata*, 37, 307–316.

Montejano, L. (1992). Recognizing sets by means of some of their sections. *Manuscripta Math.*, 76, 227–239.

Montejano, L. (1993). Orthogonal projections of convex bodies and central symmetry. *Bol. Soc. Math. Mexico*, 38, 1–7.

Montgomery, D., Samelson, H., and Zippin, L. (1956). Singular points of a compact transformation group. *Annals of Math.*, 63, 1–9.

Natterer, F. (1986). *The Mathematics of Computerized Tomography.* BG Tuebner, Stuttgart, and John Wiley & Sons Ltd.

Nonlinear Waves. (1974). (Eds. S. Leibovich and A. R. Seebass) Cornell University Press, Ithaca – London.

Novikov, S. P. (1982). The Hamiltonian formalism and multivalued analogue of Morse theory. *Russian Math. Surveys*, 37, 1–56.

Orlovskii, D. G. (1990). On a problem of determining the parameter of an evolution equation. *Differential Equations*, 26, 1201–1207.

Pekmen, U. (1995). On the dual frames of the curves on the dual sphere. *Journal of Faculty of Science Ege University*, 18, 19–25.

Petty, C. M. and McKinney, J. R. (1987). Convex bodies with circumscribing boxes of constant volume. *Portugal. Math.*, 44 (4), 447–455.

Pignoni, R. (1991). On surfaces and their contours. *Manuscripta Mathematica*, 72 (3), 223–250.

Pogorelov, A. V. (1973). *Extrinsic Geometry of Convex Bodies.* Transl. Math. Monographs, 35, AMS, Providence.

Pointet, F. (1997). Separation of hypersurfaces. *Journal of Geometry*, 59, 114–124.

Prilepko, A. I. (1992). Selected questions on the inverse problems in mathematical physics. In: *Conditionally Well-Posed Problems in Mathematical Physics and Analysis.* Nauka, Novosibirsk, 151–162 (in Russian).

Rogers, C. A. (1965). Sections and projections of convex bodies. *Portugal Math.*, 24, 99–103.

Schneider, R. (1970). Über eine Integralgleichung in der Theorie der konvexen Körper. *Mathem. Nachrichten*, 44, 55–75.

Sharafutdinov, V.A. (1992). *Integral Geometry of Tensor Fields.* VSP, Utrecht.

Spivak, M. D. (1990). *The joy of TEX.* Amer. Math. Society, Providence.

Süss, W. (1932). Zusammensetzung von Eikörpern und homothetische Eiflächen. *Tôhoku Math. Journal*, 35, 47–50.

Szczarba, R. M. (1964). On tangent bundles of fiber spaces and quotient spaces. *Amer. Journal of Math.* 84, 685–697.

Tikhonov, I. V. and Eidel'man, Yu. S. (1994). Questions of the well-posedness of direct and inverse problems for an evolution equation of special type. *Math. Notes*, 56, 99–113.

Tuy, H. K. (1983). An inversion formula for cone beam reconstruction. SIAM Journ. Math., 43, 546–551.

Znamenskii, S. V. (1985). Strong linear convexity. I. Duality of spaces of holomorphic functions. *Siberian Math. J.*, 26, 331–341.

Znamenskii, S. V. (1990). Tomography in the space of analytical functionals. *Soviet Math. Dokl.*, 312, 1037–1040.